www.fleshandbones.com

The international community for medical students and instructors. Have you joined?

For students

- Free MCQs to test your knowledge
- Online support and revision help for your favourite textbooks
- Student reviews of the books on your reading lists
- Download clinical rotation survival guides
- Win great prizes in our games and competitions

The great online resource for everybody involved in medical education

For instructors

- Download free images and buy others from our constantly growing image bank
- Preview sample chapters from new textbooks
- Request inspection copies
- Browse our reading rooms for the latest information on new books and electronic products
- Secure online ordering with prompt delivery, as well as full contact details to order by phone, fax or post

Log on and register FREE today

fleshandbones.com – an online resource for medical instructors and students

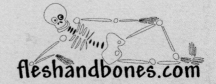

fleshandbones.com

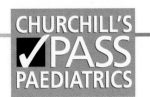

Clinical Paediatrics for Postgraduate Examinations

Commissioning Editor: Ellen Green
Project Development Manager: Jim Killgore
Project Manager: Frances Affleck
Designer: George Ajayi
Illustrator: Graeme Chambers

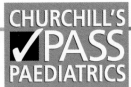

Clinical Paediatrics for Postgraduate Examinations

THIRD EDITION

Terence Stephenson
BSc BM BCh DM FRCP(UK) FRCPCH
Professor of Child Health, Queen's Medical Centre,
Nottingham

Hamish Wallace
MD FRCPCH FRCP(Edin)
Consultant Paediatric Oncologist, Royal Hospital
for Sick Children, Edinburgh

Angela Thomson
BSc MBChB MRCP(UK) MRCPCH
Specialist Registrar in Paediatrics, Royal Hospital
for Sick Children Yorkhill, Glasgow

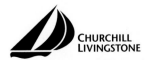

CHURCHILL
LIVINGSTONE

EDINBURGH LONDON NEW YORK PHILADELPHIA ST LOUIS SYDNEY TORONTO 2002

CHURCHILL LIVINGSTONE
An imprint of Elsevier Science Limited

First edition 1991
  Reprinted 1991
  Reprinted 1993 (twice)
Second edition 1995
  Reprinted 1996
  Reprinted 1998
Third edition 2002

ISBN 0443070415

British Library Cataloguing in Publication Data
A catalogue record for this book is available from the British Library

Library of Congress Cataloging in Publication Data
A catalog record for this book is available from the Library of
Congress

Note
Medical knowledge is constantly changing. Standard safety
precautions must be followed, but as new research and clinical
experience broaden our knowledge, changes in treatment and drug
therapy may become necessary or appropriate. Readers are advised
to check the most current product information provided by the
manufacturer of each drug to be administered to verify the
recommended dose, the method and duration of administration, and
contraindications. It is the responsibility of the practitioner, relying
on experience and knowledge of the patient, to determine dosages
and the best treatment for each individual patient. Neither the
Publisher nor the authors assumes any liability for any injury and/or
damage to persons or property arising from this publication.

your source for books,
journals and multimedia
in the health sciences
www.elsevierhealth.com

The
publisher's
policy is to use
**paper manufactured
from sustainable forests**

Printed in China by RDC Group Limited

Contents

Contents

Preface

This book has been inspired by our experience both in teaching doctors for paediatric postgraduate examinations and our own experience in passing them. This book is not a short textbook of paediatrics but a guide to the clinical examination of children. The format is specifically designed to aid revision for the clinical parts of the MRCPCH and DCH and where possible the requirements for success in these examinations have been stated. There are, by the constraints of a book that is intended to be a constant companion, some omissions, but we have tried to cover all the areas which we consider are important.

We hope that this book will appeal not only to those paediatricians entering higher medical training but also to doctors in general and community practice who have a special interest in child health.

T.S.
H.W.
A.T.

Acknowledgements

We thank the following for helpful comments: Louise Bath, Paul Eunson, Peter Gillett, Chris Kelnar, Tom Marshall, Helen Anderson, Gill Wilson and Sue Waring.

Introduction

The clinical examination in the second part of the MRCPCH exam is one of the most difficult hurdles that any paediatrician in training must face. Likewise, most candidates who fail the DCH exam do so on the clinical part. Approximately 1000–1200 candidates attempt the MRCPCH each year and 700 the DCH. A recent publication stated that 'examiners at the Royal Colleges have been dismayed by the increasing number of candidates who lacked the essential clinical skills that ought to have been gained during their undergraduate training'.

Many candidates feel that these exams are too artificial, merely test the ability to pass an exam, and are unrelated to the skills required on the ward and in the outpatient department. However, the exam is designed to test the basic clinical skills of using symptoms and signs to arrive at a diagnosis and is, on the whole, fair and not esoteric, particularly now that it is also conducted in busy provincial centres. The exam is not a game. Good candidates may fail but poor candidates rarely pass. Nevertheless, all exams are artificial and the aim of the book is to show you how to improve your technique in the unusual and demanding setting. Whilst there are many aids to passing postgraduate exams in adult medicine, there is no satisfactory guide to the clinical parts of the MRCPCH and DCH exams – which is why we wrote this book.

MEMBERSHIP OF THE ROYAL COLLEGE OF PAEDIATRICS AND CHILD HEALTH

The rules governing the MRCPCH and the MRCP(UK) Part II Paediatric option have changed substantially since 1998 and previous editions of the regulations do not apply to any examinations taken after May 2001. Therefore, if in any doubt, consult the RCPCH (see below). Since May 1999, the RCPCH has been operating its own Part I MCQ examination and no MRCP(UK) Part I Paediatric option is now available. Those who passed Part I prior to 1999 can opt for either the MRCPCH or MRCP(UK) diploma if they are successful in Part II. The Part II Paediatric option is a joint MRCPCH/MRCP(UK) examination until 2003. The Paediatric option of the MRCP(UK) Part II will cease after 2003. It is unlikely that there will be major changes to the clinical or oral examinations until 2004 at the earliest.

The Part I examination for the MRCPCH contains multiple choice questions on both basic science and clinical disorders. Areas of basic science which are particularly important for the Paediatric Part I are genetics, embryology, fetal and child physiology, growth and development, and child and family psychology. There is no longer negative marking in Part I for incorrect answers.

To qualify for the written section of the second part of the paediatric MRCPCH, you must have passed the Part I (multiple choice examination) of the MRCPCH(UK) or the paediatric Part I of the MRCP(UK) of one of the three United Kingdom colleges, unless holding one of the diplomas giving exemption from Part I (contact the RCPCH). Candidates will be able to take the Part II written examination at any time after they have passed the Part I examination. Exactly the same paper is used at a given sitting, whether in London, Edinburgh, Glasgow, Belfast or elsewhere in the world.

Since May 2001, the RCPCH has changed the examination regulations so that the written and clinical sections of the Part II MRCPCH are effectively separate examinations. Previously, the clinical was taken 6 weeks after the written examination. Now, the candidate who is successful in the written exam can defer the clinical examination. Moreover, if a candidate passes the written part but fails the clinical, the candidate does not necessarily need to re-sit the whole examination. Provided the clinical is passed within three attempts and within 2 years of the written part, the written examination does not need to be retaken. However, both the written and clinical sections of Part II must be passed within 7 years of passing Part I, otherwise Part I must be retaken.

To qualify for the clinicals of the second part of the paediatric MRCPCH, you must have passed the written section of Part II and have been fully registered for at least 18 months (at the time you undertake the clinical exam). When you take the clinical examination, you will, therefore, be at least $2\frac{1}{2}$ years from graduation, irrespective of which country you graduated in, *preferably* with a minimum of 18 months of paediatric emergency care. *Preferably*, 6 of these 18 months should be in a post undertaking management of unselected paediatric emergencies. Because there is no system for the RCPCH approving overseas posts, the only *compulsory* requirement is that at least 12 months should be spent in posts involving the care of paediatric emergencies within the last 5 years before the clinical examination. Candidates will be allowed a maximum of three attempts at the Part II clinicals within a 2-year period of passing the written exam. This 2-year period will be known as the Oral and Clinical Registration Period. Candidates who exhaust all three attempts or come to the end of their Oral and Clinical Registration Period will be required to re-enter the Part II written examination.

There is no evidence that the clinical examination is easier in one or other of the colleges. The pass rate remains remarkably consistent but varies by a small amount between each college on every sitting and no one college has a consistently higher or lower pass rate.

The Part II written examination takes place in the UK, Hong Kong, Kuwait, Malaysia, Oman, Singapore and Saudia Arabia. The Part II written exam consists of three papers: detailed case histories ('grey cases'), data interpretation and photographic material. All three sections carry approximately equal weight. To pass the written section, it is not necessary to obtain a pass mark in each of the three papers, so long as the total mark is a pass. Candidates who pass the Part II written will be eligible to enter the Part II clinical exam. The previous concept of the written section of the exam being marked out of 20, with a mark of 10 or more being considered a pass, is now irrelevant. The pass mark is not necessarily 10. If you pass the written exam, whatever the pass mark, you proceed to the clinical exam and then pass or fail the clinical exam on the criteria set out below. There is no longer the option of carrying forward a bare fail in the written (formerly 9/20) which can be compensated for in the clinical. Several books have been published giving advice on the written part of the MRCPCH.

The Part II clinical examinations are held in the UK, Hong Kong, Kuwait, Malaysia, Oman and Singapore. The clinicals for the MRCPCH examination consist of three parts which are marked independently of each other. They are the long case, the short cases and the oral, and they are usually conducted in this order. To make marking as fair as possible, each candidate is examined by a different pair of examiners for each of the three parts. Moreover, the examiners are not aware of:

● how many attempts you have previously had at the clinical exam
● your performance in the written exam
● your marks in the other sections of the clinical exam.

Each part of the clinical section is marked by the two examiners independently. A 'closed marking' system is employed, as follows:

8 Outstanding
7 Very good
6 Good
5 Pass
4 Bare pass
3 Bare fail
2 Fail
1 Bad fail
0 Abysmal

Each examiner will award one overall mark for the long case, two overall marks for the short cases (one mark for each 15-minute period conducted by each examiner) and one overall mark for the four topics covered in the oral examination. Each candidate therefore receives a total of eight separate marks (each scored out of eight) from the examiners they have seen on the day.
    A candidate will fail the examination if:

● he or she records three bare fails or lower in the eight mark sheets
● he or she records two outright fails or lower from separate examiners.

Therefore, a candidate can bare fail any two of the eight marks and still pass. About 50–70% of candidates pass the clinical at any one sitting. There is no preset quota.
    The three parts of the clinical exam are described below.

THE LONG CASE

The long case is to test the ability of the candidate:

● to take a detailed history from the child or relative
● to perform a full systematic examination, including standard testing of urine (rectal and vaginal examinations are *not* to be made even if clinically relevant)
● to have asked what investigations the child has undergone and to use the information obtained to arrive at a differential diagnosis, a problem list and a plan for management.

Candidates are allowed 1 hour for this and must then present their findings and interpretation in a succinct and clear manner and be able to elicit at the bedside the physical signs which they claim to have found. The examiners spend 20 minutes with candidates, who may also be asked to discuss the laboratory reports and X-rays. Candidates are expected to be able to suggest further relevant investigations *if these would be required in normal clinical practice*. Wildly invasive or inappropriate investigations for a minor clinical problem show inexperience and poor judgement. Candidates may be asked the plan of management, the impact on child development and the social and domestic implications of the diagnosis. They may also be asked what information should be given to the child or parents. Approximately 15 minutes are devoted by the examiners to testing history and physical signs. The last 5 minutes will be spent testing communication skills by asking candidates to explain some aspect of diagnosis, treatment or prognosis to the child or parent, with the examiners observing. Candidates are expected to 'role play' as if they were a registrar in outpatients, speaking to a parent and child, as follows:

1. Re-introduce yourself. Make eye contact with the parents and child, not the examiners. Use the child's first name.
2. Ask the parents whether they are happy for you to discuss the child's problem in front of the child, unless a pre-verbal infant.
3. Speak in lay language. Avoid abbreviations and technical terms. Be sensitive about issues such as genetic inheritance, malignancy, puberty, disability and survival if an older child is present.
4. Tell the family briefly what area you are going to discuss (introductory summary), then say it, and then tell them again (brief re-iteration of 'take home message').
5. Ask the parents whether they have any questions about what you have said.

You may not be allowed to cover all of this but you should know the principles of good communication with families.

Example

Examiner: 'Please explain to the parents of Amy (a 13-month-old girl) what the lumbar puncture which you have suggested involves.'

Candidate (speaking to and looking at parents): 'Hello again. I am Dr Miles and I'm just going to explain about one of the special tests which your baby may need. This is called a lumbar puncture – you may have heard of it?'

Parents: 'Yes, it's a bit frightening.'

Candidate: 'There's no need to worry. We use this test to obtain a few drops of fluid from around the spinal cord. We can then test this fluid in the laboratory. We will put cream on first to numb the skin over Amy's lower back and then insert some local anaesthetic – just like the dentist uses. The needle is very fine, similar to the needles she has had for blood tests in the past. We do not routinely put children to sleep – a complete general anaesthetic – for lumbar puncture because it is usually fairly quick and, with the local anaesthetic, painless. However, because we cannot explain to such a young child what we are doing, it will be necessary to hold her tightly and she may cry then. But just to recap, she will not be crying because of pain, but just because she is being held. Is there anything you want to ask me about what I have just said?'

Parents: 'Can we stay with her?'

Candidate: 'You can be present if you wish but do not feel you must be if it will upset you more. You can give Amy a cuddle immediately afterwards. Can you briefly say back to me your understanding of what we have just covered?'

Examiner: 'Thank you Dr Miles. Time is up. Please wait outside for the next part of your exam.'

Examiners exit stage left!

Candidates who struggle with this test of communication (particularly overseas candidates) do so not because of a lack of knowledge, or poor English, but either because they are not used to explaining aspects of paediatric medicine to families or because they are too embarrassed to role play. Too many candidates speak to the examiners in medical jargon, effectively excluding the parents, rather than talking to the parents in simple, plain English. If this is the case, the candidate loses easy marks.

THE SHORT CASES

The short cases are where most people fail and it is principally with these in mind that this book was written. Unlike the long case, in which there is a little time in which to collect one's thoughts after examining the patient, the short cases are conducted in the presence of the examiners to allow them to assess technique. The candidate must decide quickly what is wrong with the child and it is this ability to gently, quickly and correctly elicit physical signs and rapidly interpret them which the short cases are designed to test. The time allotted for short cases is 30 minutes; usually each examiner questions the candidate for 15 minutes while the other examiner marks. A bell may sound after 15 minutes to indicate that they should change roles, but this sequence is sometimes altered by individual examiners. The examiners will both have seen the cases before and agreed the physical signs, how difficult they are to elicit and whether it is appropriate to expect a new specialist registrar to be able to detect the signs. The examiners aim to use the short cases to assess the candidate on at least four systems, almost always including a developmental assessment. You may be asked to examine an entirely normal child. Newer techniques involving the use of mechanical aids, such as cardiopulmonary resuscitation models, videos, etc., may be used. Begin each short case by introducing yourself. Try to talk to the child as much as possible. Get down to the child's level and place the child in the position you want. Keep a young child on the parent's lap if possible. This is when a well-rehearsed, swift technique for each system, for syndromes and for developmental assessment will stand you in good stead. Candidates must clean their hands between examining patients.

The examination of a short case is frequently introduced by a piece of history, e.g. the examiner might simply say: 'Look at this child and tell me what you notice', or, alternatively: 'This young girl has become cyanosed over the last few months. Why do you think this might be?' The first question is all-embracing and you should refer to Chapter 11 on common exam syndromes for advice on how to cope with this type of question. However, examiners are encouraged by the colleges to introduce the case in order that the examination bears some similarity to real clinical practice, in which a child is rarely examined 'blind'. The second type of question is therefore an invitation to show that you can examine the relevant parts quickly, as you would have to do in a busy clinic, and step outside the restraints of a single system examination.

This difficult skill of 'rationalized examination' presumes as an essential prerequisite that you know the differential diagnosis of common physical signs. For example, if you do not know that the differential of a lump in the neck includes a lymphoma, you will not automatically offer to examine for hepatosplenomegaly and will be marked down compared with a candidate who does and can explain why. In order to convey this appearance of being able to 'think on your feet', we strongly recommend that you familiarize yourself with the lists of differential diagnoses we have provided in this book. These are also essential for the oral examination.

Examiners use three common patterns of assessment:

- full system examination (e.g. 'Examine the child's cardiovascular system')
- specific task (e.g. 'Palpate the child's precordium and listen to the heart')
- simple observation (e.g. 'Observe the child on the mother's knee and tell me what you observe').

The candidate who is given a specific task should perform this. If asked to palpate the abdomen, do not begin by examining the hands. Candidates will *not* be penalized for following instructions. However, after examining the abdomen, always offer to examine other relevant parts. Candidates will not be penalized when children become unhappy or upset during examination, provided this is not the result of the candidate's technique.

We have tried throughout the text to suggest a method for approaching a child with a common symptom or sign which allows you to examine the relevant parts in the most efficient way. This is how experienced doctors work in practice. This method stems from considering the differential diagnosis of that symptom or sign and then looking for or excluding other physical signs and thereby narrowing the differential. However, it is clearly impossible for us to cover every case which might arise in a postgraduate paediatric exam (see Boxes 1.1–1.3 for a list of cases seen by candidates whom we have recently examined), and this book is therefore about form as much as content. Perfect the habit of thinking through the following sequence so that this process is second nature even when you are confronted by a situation which we have not covered:

- differential diagnosis
- examine relevant parts
- exclude alternative diagnoses
- final diagnosis.

We have selected the 'common' short and long cases at the end of each chapter from our own experience of organizing clinical exams. Obviously, most of the children are requested to attend some time in advance, so they are likely to be children with chronic diseases and signs which do not fluctuate. However, a child with a long and complex history and virtually no physical signs may still make an excellent long case. Finally, do not be surprised to see children with acute conditions in the exam; cases may have

---

Box 1.1 Typical long cases recently encountered in the clinical part of the MRCPCH examination

A chromosome deletion syndrome
Bronchopulmonary dysplasia
Cerebral palsy
Chronic asthma
Cystic fibrosis
Down's syndrome with a ventricular septal defect
Hydrocephalus
Marfan's syndrome
Moya Moya syndrome
Nephrotic syndrome
Neurofibromatosis type I
Newly diagnosed diabetic
Ulcerative colitis and Crohn's disease

Box 1.2 Typical short cases in the clinical part of the MRCPCH examination

2-year-old with cataract
Acute arthritis
Asphyxiating thoracic dystrophy
Bulbar palsy
Café-au-lait spots
'Catch 22' syndrome
Clubbing
Developmental assessment of a normal 3-year-old
Di George's syndrome
Diabetic lipodystrophy
Duchenne's muscular dystrophy
Friedreich's ataxia
Goitre
Goldenhar's syndrome
Hemiplegia
Henoch–Schönlein purpura
Hepatosplenomegaly
Horner's syndrome
How old is this child (2 years)?
Infantile eczema
Klippel–Feil syndrome
Limp
Nephrostomy
Neurofibromatosis type I
Noonan's syndrome
Oculocutaneous albino
Optic atrophy
Osteogenesis imperfecta
Pneumonia
Portal hypertension
Ptosis
Pulmonary stenosis
Repaired coarctation
Repaired Fallot's
Russell–Silver syndrome
Scoliosis
Splenomegaly and anaemia
Strabismus
Tracheostomy for congenital haemangioma
VACTERL syndrome
Ventricular septal defect
VIth nerve palsy
VIIth nerve palsy

to be found at short notice from the wards. Moreover, the Royal Colleges have emphasized the need to make the exam a realistic test of common paediatric problems and not just a catalogue of the esoteric.

The assessment of a short case by a candidate can be made at three levels. If you are certain of the diagnosis, don't 'beat about the bush'. For example: 'This child has von Gierke's disease.' This response scores maximum marks if you are right, but if you are wrong you get no marks for 'rough work'. So, if you are less confident of your diagnosis, an appropriate statement might be: 'The abnormal findings were a very large liver, palpable kidneys, doll's

Box 1.3 Some oral topics from recent MRCPCH examinations

A 3-year-old has polyuria and polydipsia: what would you do?
APLS scenarios (e.g. arrhythmias)
Apnoea of prematurity
Blue baby
Bronchopulmonary dysplasia
Calcium metabolism
Calorie requirements at different ages
Classification of epilepsy
Coma
Desaturated infant on a ventilator
Discuss a 3-month-old with vomiting
Discuss management of a 12-year-old with headache
Education of a new diabetic
Ethical dilemmas (e.g. parents do not wish for resuscitation of very preterm
infant; cardiac surgery in Down's syndrome; disclosure of sexual abuse)
Fetal circulation
Hookworm
Hydrocephalus
Immunization schedules and contraindications
Jaundice
Kawasaki's disease
Malaria
Management of an 8-year-old with abdominal pain
Management of diabetic ketoacidosis
Meningococcal sepsis
Microcephaly
Mycobacteria
Neonatal resuscitation
Neonatal vitamin D and calcium requirements
O_2 dissociation curve
Petechiae in a neonate
Recent advances in paediatric research
Screening for cystic fibrosis and hypothyroidism
Seizures
Statistics
Stridor
The impact of molecular biology
Toddler diarrhoea, constipation and soiling
Vaginal bleeding in 3-year-old
What would you do about a baby born with ambiguous genitalia?

face and short stature. This is consistent with a glycogen storage disease.'
Even if your interpretation is wrong, you will still gain marks if the physical
signs are correct. Thirdly, if you cannot fit the signs together to make a
diagnosis, the best approach is to list the important negative and positive
findings. For example: 'There is a 10 cm, smooth, non-tender liver and both
kidneys are also palpable.' You may then be asked to commit yourself to a
diagnosis, but this is better than overconfidently plumping for a diagnosis
initially when the signs obviously did not fit, especially if it is the wrong
diagnosis. Whichever approach you adopt, you should state the summary of
your findings succinctly, clearly and confidently. Many candidates are
unsure whether to inform the examiners of physical signs as they elicit them
or to wait until they have completed their examination. Our advice is to

wait until you have completed your examination before speaking, except in the case of the developmental examination when it is important to talk as you are going along. In this way we believe you will make fewer errors and will always gain the examiners' full attention.

If you find no abnormalities, say so. Do not invent signs, as sins of commission are worse than sins of omission. Similarly, if you are very uncertain of a physical sign, e.g. whether a spleen is palpable, then it is better to be confident and say: 'The spleen is not palpable', rather than 'I think the spleen may possibly be just palpable.'

For some short cases, you will be asked only the diagnosis and to demonstrate the physical signs. However, some examiners may ask a supplementary question about relevant investigations to confirm the diagnosis, appropriate follow-up, etc.

It is said that the more short cases you see, the more likely you are to pass. While it is true that if you are on your sixth case, you are probably doing well, the converse is not true. Some 'short' cases are in fact very complex or involve more than one system and if you have only seen three difficult cases, but got them all right, you are just as likely to pass. Few candidates see more than four or five short cases. Each candidate should ideally be examined on every major system of the body (heart, chest, abdomen and a part of the CNS), usually implying a minimum of four cases, unless examination of a particular system has already been covered in the long case. In this situation, other systems will be assessed (e.g. skin, locomotor, endocrine). Most candidates fail the short cases because of a lack of technique rather than a lack of knowledge. Alternatively, they may fail because of inadequate anticipation of what type of cases to expect. This book should help with both of these pitfalls, but clearly there is no substitute for practising on the wards under exam conditions, with either a fellow candidate or a registrar taking the part of the examiner. Short cases which candidates frequently perform poorly on are examination of the eyes, examination of the motor system and developmental examination.

ORAL EXAMINATION

The oral examination is to test depth and breadth of knowledge and reasoning power. It lasts 20 minutes and the candidate is questioned by each examiner in turn. Be prepared to be asked what recent interesting articles have caught your eye in the paediatric journals. The viva topics are divided into two sections. The examiners are encouraged by the RCPCH to test all candidates on the management of acute emergencies and communication skills/ethics. At least two other topics will be selected, one from Section A and one from Section B:

● *Section A*
  1. Compulsory – management of emergencies
  plus one from:
  2. Diagnostic problems
  3. Planning management of chronic disease
  4. Recent literature including new developments.
● *Section B*
  1. Compulsory – communication skills and ethics
  plus one from:
  2. Physiology and pathophysiology
  3. Psychology; social and behavioural paediatrics
  4. Clinical research or audit/resource management/statistics.

Clinical paediatrics for postgraduate exams

Remember that under the broad headings of 'diagnostic problems', 'planning management of chronic disease' and 'physiology and pathophysiology', you could be expected to discuss the following:

- basic principles of medicine
- applied anatomy, pharmacology and biochemistry
- the physiological basis of disease processes
- basic microbiology
- nutrition
- immunization policy.

You are as likely to be asked about the physiological basis of cyanosis as about the management of acute asthma. There are always two facets to a child's problem. On the one hand, you may be asked about the investigation of a complex endocrine problem such as ambiguous genitalia, and on the other hand you may be expected to discuss sensibly the social and psychological aspects of a chronic paediatric condition such as cystic fibrosis. Child abuse is an example of the social side of paediatrics which is frequently asked about. Examiners are requested that one question relate to neonatology.

However, examiners are individuals and there is no uniform schedule that they must follow, although it is recommended that each examiner covers two different subjects. Do not be afraid to say you do not know. There is nothing more detrimental than allowing yourself to be drawn into a subject about which you know very little. No examiner expects you to know everything, but some will be only too happy to plumb the depths of your ignorance. It is clearly far better to take your chances with another topic than to press on with one about which you know little.

Finally, be prepared for the examiner who invites you to talk about a subject that interests you. This is a great chance to control proceedings and show how widely read you are. Examiners are advised not to persist on a subject about which candidates show little knowledge or, conversely, on a topic on which they are extremely well rehearsed. Some advice on oral exam technique is given in the final chapter. Again, practice makes perfect.

DIPLOMA IN CHILD HEALTH

The Diploma in Child Health (DCH) of the Royal College of Paediatrics and Child Health is held twice a year, with about 350 candidates sitting the examination on each occasion. The pass rate is approximately 65%. The examination is also held in Hong Kong. The DCH, MRCGP and MRCPCH in Paediatrics are all acceptable qualifications for registration on the General Practice Child Health Surveillance List. There is also a DCH awarded by the Royal College of Physicians and Surgeons of Glasgow and a DCH awarded by the Royal College of Physicians of Ireland. Both are principally taken by overseas candidates. The Diploma of Community Child Health (DCCH), previously organized by the Royal College of Physicians of Edinburgh, the Faculty of Public Health Medicine of the Royal College of Physicians of London and the Royal College of General Practitioners, has disappeared.

The DCH is designed to give recognition of competence in the care of children to general practitioner vocational trainees, clinical medical officers and trainees in specialties allied to paediatrics. It is also suitable as a preliminary examination for junior doctors training to be paediatricians before they attempt the more difficult MRCPCH(UK). The examination is not designed to test detailed knowledge of inpatient care of children, nor minutiae of management of rare conditions, but the philosophy is that practitioners in the community should have an understanding of hospital paediatrics in order to know when to refer and what to expect. In addition, hospital paediatricians should have a good understanding of community services. The aim is to test primary care paediatrics and the following areas are particularly emphasized in the syllabus:

- Diagnosis, management, epidemiology and prevention of common acute and chronic medical, surgical and psychological disorders in childhood.
- Principles of child health surveillance, variants of normal growth and development and minor abnormalities and their management. Candidates are expected to understand the organizational and teamwork aspects of child health surveillance and primary care and the role of other professionals and of the parent-held record.
- Knowledge of screening programmes (such as those for phenylketonuria, hypothyroidism, cystic fibrosis and haemoglobinopathies) is expected.
- The candidate should be able to demonstrate clinical skills in examination of the newborn and young infant, in particular competence in examining the hips and testes and measuring head circumference and length. Candidates should understand how pre- and perinatal care affects the subsequent progress of the infant and be able to describe the care of the normal newborn, including advice in 'lay language' for new parents on common issues such as breast- and bottle-feeding, normal bowel habit, sleep patterns, weaning. Some simple understanding of genetic counselling would also be expected.
- Knowledge of infant feeding and nutrition and the recognition and treatment of iron deficiency anaemia.
- Detailed knowledge of all aspects of immunization with all vaccines available in the UK.
- Competence in the physical and developmental examination of the infant towards the end of the first year of life is also very important. The candidate must be able to recognize serious deviations from normal development, significant features in the history suggestive of hearing loss, be able to examine the eardrums, perform a distraction test and perform visual screening tests. Candidates should also be able to take a developmental history and discuss the development of the child at any age up to 5 years, although not necessarily to do a detailed developmental assessment. The assessment and long-term management of children with disabling conditions are emphasized.
- Ability to measure height, using approved technique and equipment.
- Knowledge of behavioural problems in the physically normal child and how to advise on simple problems such as bed-wetting, sleep problems and feeding problems.
- The principles of cooperation with social services agencies, adoption and fostering and legislation relevant to children.
- Familiarity with the role of the school doctor in educational and other problems in normal and special schools.
- Knowledge of the various types and presentations of child abuse and also principles of accident prevention in the home and in the community.

It can be seen that the DCH examination concentrates on the promotion of child health, health education, immunization and screening procedures, infant feeding and nutrition and the effects of the social environment on child health, including accidents and child abuse.

Prospective candidates must have been medically qualified for at least 18 months. At least 6 months' experience in the care of children (in hospital, in the community or in general practice) is recommended, but not mandatory. Candidates are asked for details of their previous experience but this information is not shown to examiners.

The examination has written and clinical parts. Candidates who have passed the MRCP(UK) Part I examination (Paediatric option), MRCPI Part I examination (Paediatric option) or MRCPCH Part I within the last 7 years are exempt from Paper I of the DCH written exam. The written part consists of two papers:

- *Paper I* has 60 multiple choice questions for which 2 hours are allowed. Each question has an initial stem and five options, any or all of which may be true or false. There is no negative marking. An incorrect answer and 'don't know' both score zero. Paper I is marked initially and candidates must gain sufficient marks in this to go forward to the clinical section. The marks for this paper will not be used in the assessment of the overall result, but the paper acts as a screen to eliminate those candidates who have no chance of passing the examination as a whole. Approximately 80% of candidates pass Paper I. Paper II is not even marked if the candidate is eliminated due to insufficient marks in Paper I. Paper II is marked out of 10 with a pass mark of 5, but compensation from the clinicals is permissible.
- *Paper II* (3 hours) has 10 'short notes' questions and two case commentaries. The 10 'short notes' questions account for 50% of the total marks in this written paper and the case commentaries each count for 25% of the total marks in this paper.

Examples of short notes questions in Paper II
- Details of the current UK immunization schedule, e.g. contraindications to whooping cough vaccine
- Commoner surgical problems, e.g. symptoms and signs of intussusception
- Breaking bad news, e.g. neonatal diagnosis of Down's syndrome, diagnosis of cerebral palsy
- Management of behaviour problems, such as sleep disorders, temper tantrums, breath holding, food refusal, school refusal.

Answers should be approximately 100 words in length.

Examples of case commentaries in Paper II
- Communication with social services and hospital accident and emergency department about suspected physical abuse
- Communication with parents and hospital paediatrician about the provision of asthma inhalers for use at school.

Of the 3 hours allotted for this paper, approximately 1.5 hours should be spent answering the 'short notes' questions and the other 1.5 hours on the two case commentaries.

The clinical section consists of one long case and several short cases. The clinical section is designed to test the candidate's ability to take a good history, including social, behavioural and educational elements, perform a competent clinical examination, make an assessment of physical growth and development, test the special senses and assess psychiatric status if appropriate. The candidate is allowed 40 minutes for the history and examination of the long case and then spends about 20 minutes with the examiners. The examiners will assess the candidate's ability to present a succinct history, elicit any abnormal physical signs and carry out a brief developmental assessment. In addition, they will assess the candidate's ability to view the child's medical problem within the context of his/her family and wider socioeconomic background and examine the effects of the illness on physical and emotional development. The candidate may be asked to discuss management, investigations and subsequent follow-up.

Thirty minutes are allowed for the short cases and great emphasis is placed on developmental assessment, including testing of vision and hearing (see below), for which at least 10 of the 30 minutes are set aside. Each of the examiners uses approximately half the available time and, in addition to the developmental assessment, the examiners aim to assess at least three of the other major organ systems. The examiners usually introduce the short cases with a brief history and normal children may be included in the developmental assessment part of the examination. The short cases may be very short indeed and we know of one candidate who saw 10 children in 30 minutes and passed! Alternatively, you may be asked to examine several aspects of one child.

There will be three pairs of examiners and, for any given candidate, one pair of examiners will mark written Paper II, another pair will mark the long case and the third pair will mark the short case. Thus each individual candidate will be marked by three pairs of examiners. In the clinical exam, each examiner marks independently but he or she has to agree a mark on the scale of 0 to 10 for the long or the short case (0 is abysmal, 4 is a bare fail, 5 is a bare pass and 10 is outstanding). The overall result is then calculated and a pass in the clinicals and a total of 15 or more overall from written Paper II, the long case and the short case will give a pass overall. A failure in the clinicals will result in failure overall. It is not possible to compensate for a bare fail in either part of the clinical section, i.e. a candidate must pass both the long case and the short cases to pass overall. However, a bare fail in written Paper II can be compensated by a very good performance in the long or short cases. Candidates who achieve 7 or less out of 20 in the combined clinical sections may be deferred for one examination and would probably be counselled. Candidates who fail the clinical section must retake the whole of the examination, irrespective of whether they passed the written section.

The RCPCH gives specific advice on the knowledge and standards expected for the DCH, as follows:

Guidelines relating to vision, visual disorder and 'vision testing' in the DCH examination

- Background epidemiology
- History-taking
  - (i) Near acuity more important for education than distance acuity
  - (ii) Visual field defects (very rare)
  - (iii) Colour vision testing (commoner in boys)
  - (iv) Definitions of partially sighted and blind
- Observation
  - (i) Asymmetry of eyes, pupils or lids
  - (ii) Ptosis
  - (iii) Coloboma
  - (iv) Manifest squint and be able to conduct a cover test on pre-school or school age children (babies excluded)
  - (v) Abnormal eye movements, spontaneous or on testing

(vi) Opacity (red reflex)

(vii) Visually directed behaviour

(viii) Be able to test visual acuity from $3\frac{1}{2}$ years (Sheridan–Gardner or Sonksen test)

(ix) Use of parent checklist (Can your baby see?).

Guidelines for hearing testing in the DCH examination

● In the UK, distraction testing is likely to be superseded by universal newborn screening. Nevertheless, DCH candidates are still expected to be familiar with the following features of distraction testing at 6–12 months:

(i) Intensity, position, timing and source of test sound

(ii) Instructions to distracter and parent

(iii) Can child turn head?

(iv) Testing environment

(v) Pass/fail criteria and subsequent action

● Testing hearing from 18 to 30 months

● Testing hearing from $2\frac{1}{2}$ to $3\frac{1}{2}$ years

● Speech discrimination

● Distinction between screening and diagnostic tests (threshold levels of hearing, middle ear impedance, frequency audiograms, etc.).

Language development guidelines   Candidates:

● Should be able to take a history of language development

● Should be able to communicate with children of different ages

● Should be able to recognize speech disorders such as delay (commoner in boys, often associated with conductive deafness – glue ear), articulatory impairment (e.g. cerebral palsy affecting facial muscles), stammer, dysphasia (e.g. stroke), dysphonia (vocal cord palsy) and be able to discuss expressive and receptive disorders (e.g. expressive language more delayed than receptive in Down's syndrome)

● Should be aware of Makaton sign language for children with learning disabilities even with normal hearing.

Child health surveillance

● From birth to 16 years in the UK

● Criteria for a cost-effective screening test

● The meanings of screening, surveillance and assessment

● Sensitivity, specificity, false positive, false negative, positive predictive value, negative predictive value

● Legal requirements governing child care in and outside the home in the UK, including childminders, nurseries, etc.

● 'Children in need' as defined by the UK Children Act 1989

● Statementing and special educational needs

● Child abuse

● Behaviour problems

● Accident prevention

● Infant feeding, iron deficiency, failure to thrive; measure height, weight and OFC, plot on centile charts and calculate mid-parental height and target centile range

● Developmental assessment and what to do when delay detected

● UK immunization programme.

Psychiatric guidelines   Candidates should have the knowledge one would expect of a competent general practitioner or trainee general paediatrician with regard to:

- 'The terrible twos' – tantrums, feeding and sleeping difficulties
- 'The naughty boys' – aggressive or delinquent behaviour
- School refusal
- Deliberate self-harm
- Anxiety and obsessive–compulsive disorders
- Non-organic physical symptoms
- ADHD – diagnostic criteria and basic management
- Enuresis, encopresis and constipation with soiling
- Anorexia
- Autism
- Behavioural management programmes.

Detailed advice can be found on the college website (see below). This guidance would also be helpful for MRCPCH candidates.

SUMMARY

The best preparation for both the MRCPCH and the DCH examinations is undoubtedly regular practice on real cases on the wards with either a registrar or a consultant. Feedback from more senior doctors is vital to help candidates hone their skills in history-taking and physical examination. Recent changes in junior doctors' hours and the devolving of budgets to postgraduate deans have emphasized that every junior paediatric post is a training post and so every consultant is a potential teacher who should help to get their junior staff through the MRCPCH/DCH. Perhaps potential candidates should also consult with their senior colleagues on the advisability of attempting the exam at a particular time, bearing in mind the limited number of attempts allowed. In general, examiners wish the best for candidates and are not trying to catch them out, but they are aware of their responsibility for protecting children from doctors whose level of skill is not yet sufficient for more senior posts in paediatrics.

FURTHER INFORMATION

Candidates who attend examinations, whether written, clinical or oral, for the MRCPCH or DCH must be able to produce a means of identification, ideally a passport. There must be no discrepancy between the spelling, order or number of names on the original medical qualification, the examination application form and the passport. Candidates who change their name, by marriage or otherwise, must submit documentary proof of this. Further information about both the MRCPCH and the DCH can be obtained from the following address:

Royal College of Paediatrics and Child Health
50 Hallam Street
London W1W 6DE
Tel: 020 7307 5600
Fax: 020 7307 5601
Website: www.rcpch.ac.uk/exams

The website contains both information on how to apply for the examinations and also brief advice on 'Clinical examination technique in paediatrics'. Obviously this is not as good as the contents of this book! Where relevant, advice from the website has been checked for agreement with this book.

Long case

2

In the long case section of the exam candidates have 1 hour to obtain a full history and carry out an examination of the child. This is followed by a 20-minute viva with two examiners who do not usually allow time for a complete verbatim history, but instead will expect an account of the child's condition with emphasis on current problems and the impact of the child's condition on the family. The examiners will always have seen the long case prior to the candidates. The long case can be considered as being like a new patient who has recently moved to your area and is attending for the first appointment at your hospital. One of the most crucial aspects of the history is to present the story in an orderly, logical *and chronological* sequence. You must present the important positive and negative findings relevant to the child's condition. Examiners may interject at any time with questions like: 'How has this affected the child's development?' or 'What impact has this had on the rest of the family?'

One of the most important points about this part of the exam is that the 1 hour with the family goes very fast, so it is essential to practise good time management. Generally spend approximately 25 minutes on the history and 20 minutes on the examination, leaving yourself with 15 minutes to organize your thoughts, come up with a problem list and a management plan and think of possible questions the examiners may ask you. This will also allow some time if, in preparing your summary, you realize there are other questions you should have asked or other signs you should have looked for. Some candidates mistakenly believe there are certain areas they should not ask about – that they will be thought to have cheated if they ask the parents the diagnosis, the treatment or what tests the child has had. The examination is supposed to replicate, as near as possible, real paediatric practice. Practising doctors ask parents these questions all the time – it is part of the child's history – so you should ask them in the exam. Most parents are very knowledgeable about their child's condition and are sometimes up to date with the latest on the internet – they want to help you to pass. The parents are asked to answer all the questions you ask, just as they would if attending outpatients.

Common omissions in the long case are:

- Insufficient detail about the child's presenting complaints, e.g. a precise eyewitness description of the child's typical seizure (see below)
- Accepting the child's or parent's terminology without question. Candidates often accept terms such as 'wheeze', 'migraine' or 'convulsion' uncritically, only to find out from the examiners that the parent did not mean what you mean! Too late.
- The child's past and current drug treatment
- Drug side-effects
- Who administers the drug (parent, teacher, child) and using which device (e.g. inhaled drugs, self-injection, etc.)

- Blood pressure
- Height, weight and head circumference plotted on age- and sex-appropriate centile charts
- Parental heights and calculation of mid-parental height and target centile range (see p. 106) if appropriate
- Parental head circumferences if appropriate.

HISTORY (GUIDE)

The history-taking must be adapted to the child's age and level of ability. Talk to the child and get him or her on your side.

Child's first and last names

Age

Source of history (mother/father/other)

Presenting complaint
Give the presenting complaint at the time of current admission or give a brief numbered list if there are several simultaneous presenting complaints. Use the words of the person talking to you. He or she may tell you the diagnosis. If the child is not currently an inpatient, you will have to ask about current problems (there may be none if the child is currently asymptomatic) or problems discussed at the last outpatient visit.

History of presenting complaint

Chronological sequence of events
- Mode of presentation
- Sequence and duration of hospital admissions or outpatient attendances.

Management
- Investigations
- Medications
- Surgery
- Timing of complications and their management.

Checklist for important symptoms (e.g. vomiting, diarrhoea, wheeze, headaches, seizures etc.) – **don't forget!**   Time of onset, site, duration, frequency, severity, relieving/aggravating factors, seasonal variation, etc.

Past medical history

Birth history (more detail is required if it is a neonatal, developmental or genetic case)
- Antenatal problems
- Gestation and mode of delivery
- Resuscitation required
- Admitted to the neonatal unit – why?

Nutritional history
- Breast/bottle-fed – duration
- Weaning
- Current dietary intake – if relevant to complaint of older child or diabetic.

Developmental history
● Gross motor, fine motor, language and social skills – know at least four milestones for 3, 6, 9, 12 and 18 months and 2, 3 and 4 years which parents can easily answer.

Previous hospital admissions
● Including A&E attendance, outpatient, day-case surgery.

Immunization history
● If any immunizations have been omitted, ask why.

Drug history
Past and present, including full details of dose and frequency of current medication.

Allergies
Foods, medications etc.

Family history
● Have any family members had a similar illness or any other serious disorder? Genetic, metabolic, allergic and infectious illnesses may all be shared by other family members. Children may also 'learn' symptom clusters from older siblings or adults, e.g. a so-called 'migraine' may have none of the typical features on more detailed exploration.
● In particular, is there a family history of asthma, eczema, hay fever, food allergy, diabetes or epilepsy, as these are all relatively common in the general population?
● A family tree is the most useful way to communicate the information, particularly if there is a history of hereditary conditions.

Social history
● Important information should include the following: age, occupation, health, marital status, consanguinity (particularly common in Asian Muslim families), smoking habits, who lives at home, details of contact with the other parent if it is a single-parent family
● Housing – type, owned or rented, any special modifications, number of bedrooms
● Respite/family support
● Financial support
● Pets.

Education
● On Special Needs Register?
● Mainstream school +/– learning support teacher or special school
● Peer relationships
● Behaviour.

Systems enquiry
There are a few general questions which provide a useful 'screen' and the remainder are rarely necessary unless there is a chronic multisystem disease.

General screen
- Appetite
- Weight loss
- Is the child his or her usual self?
- Level of activity
- Any breathing problems
- Bowel habit
- Any recent change in behaviour or personality?

Cardiovascular
- Breathless – on exertion, slow to feed, sweaty on feeding
- Cyanotic episodes
- Squatting
- Chest pain or palpitations
- Dizzy spells or faints.

Respiratory
- Sore throat/earache
- Cough – nocturnal
- Sputum
- Breathlessness – compared with peers during games
- Frequent chest infections
- Aspiration of foreign body
- Haemoptysis.

Gastrointestinal
- Swallowing difficulties
- Vomiting or nausea
- Abdominal pain
- Diarrhoea or constipation
- Blood in stools
- Pruritus ani
- Jaundice
- Foreign travel, contacts, dietary history – if infectious disease.

Genitourinary
- Stream
- Dysuria
- Frequency
- Nocturia
- Enuresis (primary/secondary)
- Haematuria
- Menstrual history.

Neurological
- Fits, faints or funny turns
- Headaches
- Anosmia
- Visual disturbances
- Deafness, tinnitus or dizziness
- Paraesthaesia
- Weakness, clumsiness or frequent falls
- Incontinence.

Musculoskeletal
- Limp
- Joint pain or swelling
- Skin rash
- Dry mouth or ulcers
- Dry or sore eyes

● Alopecia
● Cold peripheries.

The history will guide your physical examination so concentrate on these areas when looking for signs but also complete a thorough examination. For instance, a child with developmental delay may have an incidental innocent heart murmur which the examiner would expect you to pick up.

The commonest errors by candidates during the 20 minutes with the examiners are as follows:

● An inability to provide a concise summary or formulation of the case.
● Reading the history from written notes verbatim – this is boring and shows a lack of critical thought. You should make eye contact with the examiners and present the case as you would on a ward round, emphasizing the important positive and negative points.
● Starting with the history of the presenting complaint – *always* start with a list of problems or diagnoses. Then the examiners know the child has congenital heart disease, short stature and cerebral palsy without having to wait 10 minutes to hear you say this. Remember, the examiners and the parent (and the child) already know the diagnosis and would be astonished if you didn't.
● A failure to be able to present a concise *chronological* sequence of events – from presentation to investigation, then diagnosis and treatment, followed by subsequent management, admissions, sequelae, etc.
● An inability to describe the drugs the child receives – with doses, frequency, devices and any previous side-effects.
● See the introductory chapter for advice on communicating with the family. You will usually be asked to spend the last 5 minutes with the examiner demonstrating your communication skills by 'role play' (i.e. as you would do this in a real life situation).

GENERAL ADVICE ON EXAMINING CHILDREN

First know what is normal by examining as many babies, infants, toddlers and children as possible – the abnormal will then be more obvious.

The art of examining a child requires repeated rehearsal until it becomes second nature. To look as if you have examined a child 100 times you need to do so! Efficient and slick technique will impress the examiner even though you may not necessarily detect all the abnormalities present. A guide to examining each of the systems is given in the following chapters but a few general rules, as follows, should be applied whatever the system.

1. **Introduce yourself to both the child and parent.**
2. **Ask the child's name** – if not already given it.
3. **Establish rapport with the child** – talk softly to the child during examination; do not frighten them.
4. **Inspection** – this is the key to success. Observe the child during the history as he or she may cry during the examination. Find out as much as you can from the end of the bed before you approach, touch or undress the child. Look for:

General well-being
Severity of illness
Conscious level (not to be confused with normal sleep) – know the Glasgow Coma Scale (see p. 24)
Pink/cyanosed/anaemic/jaundiced

Respiratory rate/accessory muscles and tracheal tug/audible wheeze/ stridor

Growth/nutrition; size in relation to age

Head size in relation to body

Dysmorphic features suggesting a genetic syndrome

Acquired features of underlying illness (e.g. frontal bossing of thalassaemia or hydrocephalus, clubbing of chronic respiratory or cardiac disease)

Spectacles, squint, nystagmus, roving eye movements, ptosis, sunsetting

Development

Speech

Behaviour

Posture

Spontaneous movements

Extra equipment around the bed (e.g. saturation monitor and the heart rate and current saturation, ECG monitor, oxygen mask, nebulizer or spacer, suction machine, sputum pot, continuous enteral feeding pump, intravenous lines and fluid bags, urinary catheter bag, splints, wheelchair, etc.).

5. **Keep hands warm and free of jewellery** – it may be impractical to wash hands between cases.
6. **Give clear simple instructions confidently.**
7. **Position the child appropriately** – a happy child on the mother's knee is better than a crying child at 45° on the bed, but explain your decision to the examiners.
8. **Help undress the child.**
9. **Ask about pain** – before examining.
10. **Tell the child what you are going to do** – do not ask permission, as he or she may say no. Rather, adopt a confident, assertive but sympathetic approach, e.g. 'I am going to listen to your tummy.' Listening to teddy's tummy first may win round an awkward child.
11. **Ask the parent/examiner to distract the child with a toy.**
12. **Examination is age-dependent** – young and uncooperative children require an *opportunistic* approach; this requires flexibility in your examination but presentation of your findings must be in a structured manner.
13. **Measurements** – plot height, weight, OFC on growth chart. Don't forget special centile charts for children with Down's and Turner's syndromes. Plot the parents' parameters if necessary. Don't forget to do blood pressure, urinalysis, fundoscopy and ENT examinations at the end of the examination in the long case.
14. **Appropriate equipment** – you may find it easier if familiar with your own equipment. This does not necessarily mean bringing a suitcase to the exam, rather a few toys for developmental assessment and an ophthalmoscope as a minimum.
15. **Answer the question asked** – not the one you would have liked!

Some further general rules are outlined below:

- Rectal and vaginal examinations should not be performed in any part of the MRCPCH or DCH. However, you should indicate when these would be appropriate.
- You are not expected routinely to examine the external genitalia or perianal region. If this is required, you will be specifically asked to do this.

- Use discretion when examining a pubertal or postpubertal child, but you should indicate when greater exposure of the body would be appropriate for complete examination.
- You should be able to measure the peak flow rate, know the result relates to the child's height and be able to assess inhaler technique.
- Leave potentially unpleasant tests to the end (e.g. auriscope, blood pressure, femoral pulses, hip tests).
- You should have a rough idea of the normal range of blood pressure with age and the difficulties of obtaining reliable blood pressure measurements. You are expected to be able to use a mercury sphygmomanometer and choose an appropriate cuff, but you are not expected to know how to use automated blood pressure devices.
- You should be able to direct the parents to assist in holding the child appropriately whilst the ears are examined.
- You should know how to examine the anterior nares with an auriscope.
- One of the most commonly asked questions by candidates preparing for the exam is: 'Should I give a running commentary or present my findings at the end?' This causes candidates endless stress as different examiners like different approaches. We would advise against a running commentary unless specifically asked, as it is easy to commit yourself wrongly to a physical sign before you have the complete picture. One exception to this is the developmental assessment, where commenting as you observe the child may be helpful.
- You should be able to recognize and interpret diagnostic imaging at the level of a new specialist registrar (CXR, CT, MRI, neonatal brain ultrasound, abdominal X-ray, MCUG, IVU, DMSA, MAG3, Hida scan, upper and lower GI contrast studies, plain radiology of bones and joints, isotope bone scan). You are not expected to interpret bronchograms, V/Q scans, other ultrasound scans, arteriography or arthrography.

GLASGOW COMA SCALE

Eye opening	1 = None
	2 = To pain
	3 = To speech
	4 = Spontaneous
Best motor response	1 = None
	2 = Extensor response to pain
	3 = Abnormal flexion to pain
	4 = Withdraws from pain
	5 = Localizes pain
	6 = Obeys command
Best verbal response	1 = None
	2 = Incomprehensible sounds
	3 = Inappropriate words
	4 = Appropriate words but confused
	5 = Fully orientated

Notes:
1. Maximum score = 15. Score ≤8 is serious – admit to ICU.
2. Spontaneous extensor posturing (decerebrate) scores 2 and spontaneous flexor posturing (decorticate) scores 3 on the motor scale.
3. *Modification of verbal response score for younger children:*

2–5 years	**<2 years**
1 = None	1 = None
2 = Grunts	2 = Grunts
3 = Cries or screams	3 = Inappropriate crying or unstimulated screaming
4 = Monosyllables	4 = Cries only
5 = Words of any sort	5 = Appropriate non-verbal responses (smiles, coos, cries)

SUMMARY PLAN FOR LONG CASE

History	Examination	Case summary/formulation
Name	*Each system*	1. Differential diagnosis
Age	*Do not forget:*	2. Investigations
Source	● Blood pressure	3. Problem list
PC	● Development	4. Management plan
HPC	● Fundoscopy	5. Possible questions
PMH	● Growth charts	
● Birth	● Urinalysis	
● Nutrition		
● Development		
● Immunizations		
● Previous illnesses		
Drugs		
Allergies		
FH		
SH		
● Parents/siblings		
● Housing		
● Respite/support		
● Education		
● Behaviour		
SE		

The cardiovascular system

3

This chapter presents a full account of the cardiovascular examination. However, in our experience, the candidate is usually requested only to examine a part of the system, e.g. 'feel the pulse', 'localize the apex beat' or 'listen to the heart'. You should therefore follow the examiners' instructions exactly in order to avoid antagonizing them.

INSPECTION

GENERAL

- General health, e.g. nutritional status, failure to thrive, tachypnoeic
- Dysmorphic features, e.g. Down's, Turner's, Noonan's or Williams syndrome.

FACE

Colour

Cyanosis Implies desaturated blood in the capillaries (>5 g/dL), giving the skin and mucous membranes a bluish discoloration, characteristic of right-to-left shunts within the heart or between the great arteries, or as a consequence of inadequate oxygenation of blood in the lungs. It corresponds to an arterial saturation of about 75% for a haemoglobin of 12–16 g/dL. Consequently, it can be present at a normal P_aO_2, if there is polycythaemia, or be difficult to detect if there is concomitant anaemia. It is clinically detected as follows:

- central (right-to-left shunts, cardiac or lung) – tongue
- peripheral (inadequate peripheral circulation) – nailbeds.

Pallor This is best detected in the oral mucosae, lips and conjunctivae. If associated with poor cardiac output, pulses may be weak and tissue perfusion poor.

Polycythaemia Often found in association with cyanotic congenital heart disease. These children have a high haematocrit and increased viscosity associated with an increased risk of cerebrovascular events.

Teeth
Comment on dental caries, indicating the importance of dental care as part of outpatient follow-up.

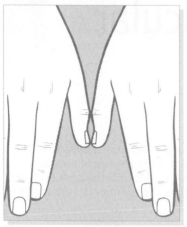
'Diamond' created by nailbeds

Not clubbed —
nailbed angle acute (Schamroth's sign)

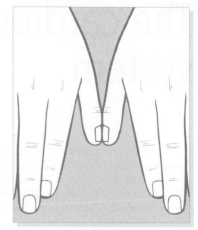
Loss of diamond

Clubbed —
loss of nailbed angle

Fig. 3.1   Finger clubbing.

HANDS

Clubbing
Increased longitudinal and lateral curvature of the nails with loss of the acute angle between the proximal part of the nail and the skin, best seen at sites of largest surface area, such as thumbs and great toes (Fig. 3.1).

Bony abnormalities
- Absent radii – VACTERL syndrome
- Absent thumbs – Holt–Oram syndrome.

Rarities
- Splinter haemorrhages and Osler's nodes of infective endocarditis
- Tuberous and tendon xanthomata of familial hypercholesterolaemia. Feel over the elbows in a hypertensive child.

CHEST

Respiratory rate

Scars (Fig. 3.2)

Asymmetry
Look from the side in the same plane as the chest for:

- anterior bulge left chest – cardiomegaly
- left parasternal heave – right ventricular hypertrophy
- visible pulsations
- Harrison's sulci – in conditions with increased pulmonary blood flow or chronic asthma.

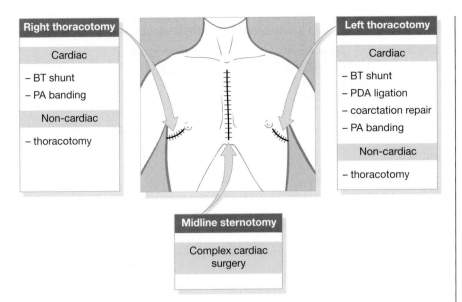

Fig. 3.2 Scars. BT, Blalock–Taussig; PA, pulmonary artery; PDA, patent ductus arteriosus.

PALPATION

PULSES

Brachial pulses

In young children the brachial pulse is the easiest to palpate. Ensure that both brachial pulses are present and equal in volume. If there is an *absent or reduced brachial pulse,* this is indicative of one of the following:

- classic left Blalock–Taussig shunt – absent left brachial pulse
- classic right Blalock–Taussig shunt – absent right brachial pulse
- left subclavian artery repair of coarctation – absent left brachial pulse
- flap aortoplasty repair of coarctation – reduced left brachial pulse
- previous cardiac catheterization – absent radial or brachial pulse
- cervical rib – either brachial pulse absent (especially on shoulder abduction)
- embolization
- congenital malformation – absent radial pulse.

Assess the following, using the right brachial pulse.

Rate Always count this over 10 seconds whilst deliberately looking at your watch. Never guess. Table 3.1 gives heart rates for healthy children. Abnormal rates could be:

- bradycardia (rare in exams)
  — junior athletes!
  — drugs (β-blockers and digoxin)
  — complete heart block
- tachycardia – sinus tachy in anxious child.

Table 3.1 Heart rates in healthy children

Age (years)	Normal range (bpm)
0–2	80–140
2–6	75–120
>6	70–110

Rhythm

Regular
- Respiratory sinus arrhythmia (universal in young children).

Regularly irregular
- Pulsus bigeminous, coupled extrasystoles (digoxin toxicity).

Irregularly irregular
- Multiple extrasystoles – common in young children, they disappear on exertion
- Atrial fibrillation
  — atrial septal defect (ASD)
  — open heart surgery or atrial surgery
  — Ebstein's anomaly of tricuspid valve
  — rheumatic mitral stenosis (immigrant children only).

Check the apical rate by auscultation for the true heart rate as small pulses may not be transmitted.

Volume

Small volume
- Pump failure – heart failure
- Shock – circulatory failure due to hypovolaemia
- Outflow obstruction – aortic stenosis (AS) or pericardial effusion.

The first two are commoner in practice, but the third is commoner in exams.

Large volume
- Anaemia
- Carbon dioxide retention
- Thyrotoxicosis (very rare).

Varying volume
- Extrasystoles
- Atrial fibrillation
- Incomplete heart block.

Character　The character of the pulse may be one of the following (see also Fig. 3.3):

- normal
- slow rising – moderate to severe aortic stenosis
- collapsing
  — aortic incompetence (AI) (rare)
  — patent ductus arteriosus (PDA) (large volume, rapid collapse – often a neonatal case)
- bisferiens – moderate aortic stenosis with severe aortic incompetence (very rare)

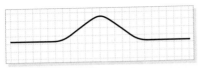

Normal

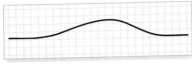

Slow rising

Moderate to severe aortic stenosis

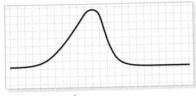

Collapsing pulse

Aortic incompetence (rare)
PDA (large volume, rapid collapse — often neonatal case)

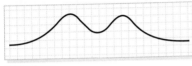

Bisferiens

Moderate aortic stenosis with severe aortic incompetence (very rare)

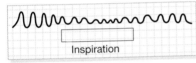

Inspiration

Pulsus paradoxus

An exaggeration of a normal phenomenon, i.e. the fall in blood pressure on inspiration.

Fig. 3.3 Character of pulses.

- pulsus paradoxus – not a paradox at all but an exaggeration of a normal phenomenon, i.e. the fall in blood pressure on inspiration. If detected, offer to check by sphygmomanometry. A paradox of greater than 15 mmHg is abnormal. Causes include:
  — pericardial effusion
  — constrictive pericarditis
  — severe airways obstruction (asthma)
  (all are very unlikely in an exam).
- rapidly rising, ill-sustained, jerky – hypertrophic obstructive cardiomyopathy (HOCM).

Femoral pulses
Absence of femoral pulses is indicative of coarctation. This can be checked at the end of the examination. Radiofemoral delay is difficult to detect in children.

Suprasternal notch
Gentle palpation will detect a thrill in aortic stenosis. AS is a fairly common

exam case and is easily missed if you press too hard, so make sure you have seen at least one case *before* the exam.

The jugular venous pressure (JVP) is generally not an important part of the paediatric cardiovascular system. It can only be measured in older children and, whilst it is elevated in right heart failure, fluid overload and pericardial tamponade, none of these is likely in the exam.

BLOOD PRESSURE

Although you are rarely asked to do this in an exam, you must say you would do it and know how to do so if you are asked to measure it! The cuff must cover at least two-thirds of the upper arm, with a bladder that completely encircles the arm. In younger children, systolic blood pressure can be approximately determined by palpation of the brachial pulses as the cuff is deflated. In older children you must listen over the brachial pulse with a stethoscope. Record the blood pressure in the right arm and note whether the child is sitting, standing or supine. It is impossible to get accurate readings when a child is crying. Win cooperation by asking the child to 'see how strong you are' and by getting him/her to watch the mercury column rise and fall. Blood pressure varies with age but a rough guide is as follows:

● mean diastolic = 55 + age in years
● mean systolic = 90 + age in years.

The upper limits of normal are (mean + 20) mmHg for diastolic and (mean + 18) mmHg for systolic.

APEX BEAT

Position
This is described as the furthest lateral and inferior position at which the finger is lifted by the cardiac impulse, and is *normally the fourth intercostal space in the midclavicular line*. Always be seen to define the position by counting down from the second rib space which lies below the second rib (opposite the manubriosternal angle). Describe its position in relation to the midclavicular line, anterior and mid-axillary lines.

The beat may be:

● Displaced to the left
 — cardiomegaly
 — scoliosis
 — pectus excavatum
● On the right side
 — congenital dextrocardia: feel for the liver (Kartagener's syndrome)
 — acquired dextroposition: heart pushed or pulled to the right
 — left diaphragmatic hernia (rare in exams)
 — collapsed lung on the right side (rare in exams).

Quality
● Sustained – with *pressure* overload in aortic stenosis
● Forceful – left ventricular hypertrophy
● Thrusting – with *volume* overload: an active large stroke volume ventricle in mitral or aortic incompetence, or left-to-right shunt

● Parasternal heave – right ventricular hypertrophy.

Thrills
The accompanying murmur is by definition at least 4/6 in intensity. Localize the site. For a *systolic thrill*:

● lower left sternal edge – ventricular septal defect (VSD)
● upper left sternal edge – pulmonary stenosis (PS).

Palpable heart sounds
A *second sound* reflects pulmonary hypertension.

NB. If you find an abnormality, think of possible causes before you listen, and what murmur you would expect to hear, e.g.:

● collapsing pulse – ?aortic incompetence
● suprasternal thrill – ?aortic stenosis.

AUSCULTATION

Listen over the four main areas of the heart whilst palpating the right brachial pulse with your left hand and in each area concentrate on:

● heart sounds
● added sounds
● murmurs.

Also present your findings in this manner, in order not to forget things.
    The four main areas are (Fig. 3.4):

● apex (and axilla if there is a murmur)
● tricuspid area

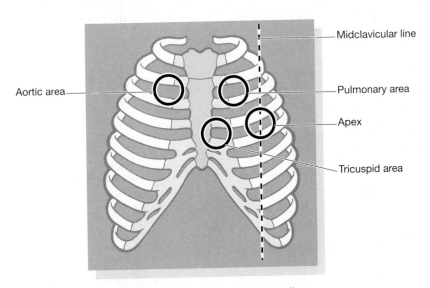

Fig. 3.4   Auscultation of praecordium.

Clinical paediatrics for postgraduate exams

- aortic area (and neck if there is a murmur)
- pulmonary area (listen over the back if there is a murmur).

Listen over the apex, first with the bell and then with the diaphragm of the stethoscope, and then continue with the diaphragm over the other areas. Always listen at the back – innocent murmurs do not radiate to the back. Murmurs of pulmonary stenosis radiate to the back. With an older, cooperative child, always listen again along the lower left sternal edge (LSE).

- Murmur loudest in expiration – left heart disease
- Murmur loudest in inspiration – right heart disease

HEART SOUNDS (Fig. 3.5)

Normal heart sounds
- First sound – sudden cessation of mitral and tricuspid flow due to valve closure
- Second sound – sudden cessation of aortic and pulmonary flow due to valve closure.

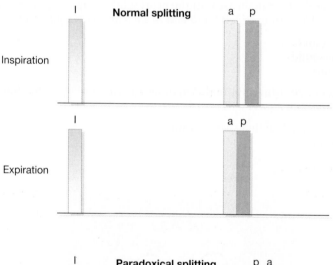

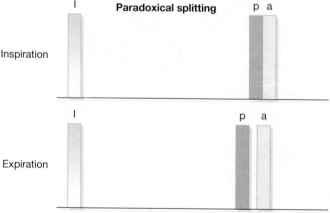

Fig. 3.5   Heart sounds. a, aortic valve; p, pulmonary valve.

Loud first sound
● ASD
● Mechanical prosthetic valve
● Mitral stenosis (MS) (very rare in paediatric exams).

Variable loudness of first sound
● Heart block
● Atrial fibrillation.

Loud second sound
This is *very important* in paediatric cardiology. If it is of normal intensity and splits normally, many important conditions are excluded.

● Increased pulmonary flow – PDA, ASD, large VSD
● Pulmonary hypertension.

Split second sound
● Universal in healthy children and widens on inspiration. Aortic closure precedes pulmonary closure
● Fixed splitting (no change with respiration) – ASD
● Widely split – ASD, PS, right bundle branch block (RBBB)
● Reversed splitting (widens on expiration) – severe AS, left bundle branch block (LBBB).

Single second sound (inaudible pulmonary component)
● Tetralogy of Fallot
● Pulmonary stenosis.

ADDED SOUNDS

Third sound
After the second sound, i.e. early diastole, low-pitched.

● Rapid ventricular filling, normal in healthy children
● Best heard with the bell over the apex
● May be confused with a split second sound or opening snap
● Heard in failure of either ventricle.

Fourth heart sound
● Never a normal finding
● Precedes first sound
● Failure of either ventricle
● Pulmonary hypertension.

Opening snap (Fig. 3.6)
● After second sound, high-pitched
● Mitral stenosis.

Ejection click (Fig. 3.6)
● After first sound, high-pitched, early systole
● Aortic or pulmonary stenosis.

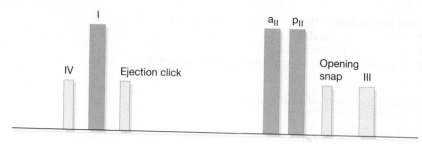

Fig. 3.6   Added heart sounds.

MURMURS

Try to define the following:

- Intensity (grades 1–6 if systolic, 1–4 if diastolic; grade 4 if thrill is palpable)
- Site where heard loudest
- Radiation
- Timing (systolic, diastolic or both)
- Duration (e.g. early diastolic or pansystolic)
- Pitch and quality (e.g. high or low, harsh or blowing)
- Changes with respiration or posture.

Remember to listen over the back (PDA, PS and coarctation).

Normal murmurs (previously called innocent or benign)
Cardiac murmurs are common in paediatrics. Accurate assessment of the child following the guidelines below will help to distinguish normal from pathological murmurs. Diagnosing a normal murmur positively rather than by exclusion will reduce unnecessary referrals and undue anxiety in the parents.

The '10 S' test of a normal murmur is as follows:

- Symptom-free
- Systolic
- Short
- Soft
- Site – heard over a small area only
- Split second sound
- Sitting/standing (i.e. varies with posture)
- Sternal depression (benign murmurs with pectus excavatum)
- Signs – no other abnormal signs, all pulses are normal
- Special tests (ECG and chest X-ray are normal).

There are basically five types of normal murmur which originate from increased flow velocity.

Still's murmur   Early soft systolic murmur heard over the lower left sternal edge. Usually grade 2 in intensity but can be louder and often has a musical or buzzing quality to it. Murmur will decrease or disappear on hyperextension. Try it in an older, cooperative child.

Pulmonary flow murmur   Soft ejection systolic murmur, usually ≤ grade 2, heard over the second left intercostal space. Rarely propagated posteriorly.

Can be confused with pulmonary flow murmur associated with ASD but there is no wide fixed splitting of second heart sound.

Venous hum   Continuous murmur with diastolic accentuation heard below right clavicle and radiating to base. Often loud, grade 3, the intensity decreases when supine and can be obliterated by gentle neck compression. Still's murmur is often also present.

Supraclavicular or carotid bruit   Best heard above the clavicles, although it transmits downwards.

Neonatal physiological peripheral artery stenosis murmur   Maximal over upper left sternal edge and usually ≤ grade 2. Radiates throughout the thorax, to both axillae and to the back. Most disappear by 6 months of age and all have gone by 12 months.

Pathological murmurs
Using the following criteria – the seven cardinal signs – it is estimated that 95% of pathological murmurs would be identified:

- Pansystolic murmur
- Intensity ≥ grade 3
- Intensity maximal at upper left sternal edge
- Posterior propagation of murmur
- Harsh quality
- Early or mid-systolic click
- Abnormal second heart sound.

Classification of pathological murmurs
- Systolic (see Table 3.2)
- Diastolic (see Table 3.3)
- Continuous (see Table 3.4).

Table 3.2 Systolic murmurs

Cause	Type	Site
Innocent flow murmur	ESM	Left sternal edge or pulmonary area
Anaemia	ESM	Left sternal edge or aortic area
VSD	PSM	Left sternal edge, fourth intercostal space
PS	ESM	Pulmonary area, left second intercostal space
ASD	ESM	Pulmonary area, left second intercostal space
Aortic stenosis or bicuspid aortic valve	ESM	Aortic area, right second intercostal space to carotids in AS AS (rare), bicuspid valve (quite common) May radiate to carotids
Coarctation	PSM	Left sternal edge and between scapulae
HOCM	Late SM	Rare
Mitral regurgitation	PSM	Apex and left axilla
Mitral valve prolapse	Late SM	Apex

ESM, ejection systolic murmur; PSM, pansystolic murmur; HOCM, hypertrophic obstructive cardiomyopathy

Table 3.3 Diastolic murmurs

Cause	Site
ASD	Tricuspid flow murmur, low-pitched over sternal edge
VSD	Mid-diastolic mitral flow murmur with large defect
Mitral stenosis (rare)	Low-pitched at apex

Table 3.4 Continuous murmurs

Cause	Site
Innocent venous hum	Below either clavicle, may disappear when lying down or with legs elevated
PDA	Below left clavicle, radiates to back
Coarctation	Left sternal edge and between scapulae

Quality
- High frequency, blowing – mitral regurgitation (MR), aortic regurgitation (AR), pulmonary regurgitation (PR)
- Low frequency, harsh – AS, PS, VSD
- Lower frequency, rumbling – MS.

A summary of murmurs is presented in Figure 3.7.

ANYTHING ELSE?

- Feel for hepatomegaly
- Femoral pulses – do this at the end when examining babies as it is unpleasant and will make them cry
- Blood pressure – say you would like to do this if you have not already done so
- Height and weight – say you would like to plot these parameters on a growth chart appropriate for age and sex.

PRESENTATION OF HEART DISEASE

ASYMPTOMATIC MURMUR

- Neonatal check
- 6-week check
- Pre-school check
- Routine check with other illness.

Commonest causes
- VSD
- ASD
- PDA
- PS
- Coarctation
- AS.

PASS ✓

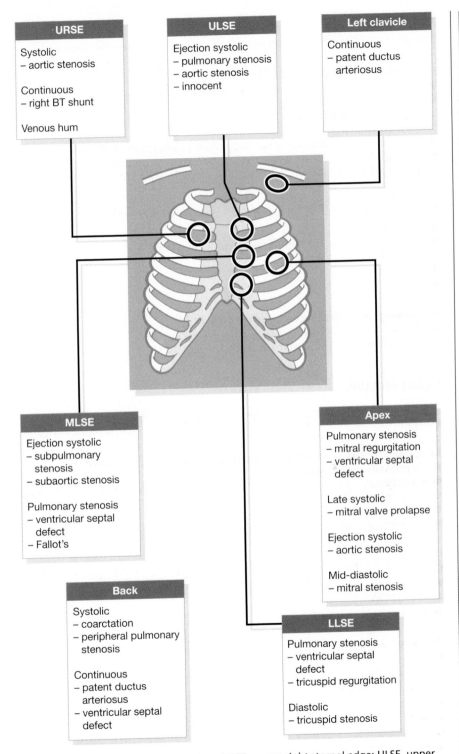

URSE

Systolic
– aortic stenosis

Continuous
– right BT shunt

Venous hum

ULSE

Ejection systolic
– pulmonary stenosis
– aortic stenosis
– innocent

Left clavicle

Continuous
– patent ductus
  arteriosus

MLSE

Ejection systolic
– subpulmonary
  stenosis
– subaortic stenosis

Pulmonary stenosis
– ventricular septal
  defect
– Fallot's

Apex

Pulmonary stenosis
– mitral regurgitation
– ventricular septal
  defect

Late systolic
– mitral valve prolapse

Ejection systolic
– aortic stenosis

Mid-diastolic
– mitral stenosis

Back

Systolic
– coarctation
– peripheral pulmonary
  stenosis

Continuous
– patent ductus
  arteriosus
– ventricular septal
  defect

LLSE

Pulmonary stenosis
– ventricular septal
  defect
– tricuspid regurgitation

Diastolic
– tricuspid stenosis

Fig. 3.7 Summary of cardiac murmurs. URSE, upper right sternal edge; ULSE, upper left sternal edge; BT, Blalock–Taussig; MLSE, mid left sternal edge; LLSE, lower left sternal edge.

CYANOSIS

The child's age at presentation is important in determining the aetiology.

Presenting in first week of life – five Ts
- Transposition of the great arteries – abnormal mixing
- Total common mixing:
  - total AV canal defect
  - truncus arteriosus
- Total pulmonary atresia – duct-dependent pulmonary circulation
- Tricuspid atresia – duct-dependent pulmonary circulation
- Tricuspid regurgitation and Ebstein's anomaly with right-to-left shunt via ASD.

Don't forget other causes of cyanosis in the neonatal period:

- respiratory
- persistant pulmonary hypertension of the newborn
- metabolic
- haematological
- sepsis.

Presenting after first week of life – two Ts
- Tetralogy of Fallot (can present earlier if very severe)
- Total anomalous pulmonary venous drainage (TAPVD).

HEART FAILURE

Less likely to be seen in an exam but you must know the causes, signs and symptoms.

Neonatal period (obstructed duct-dependent systemic circulation)
- Hypoplastic left heart syndrome
- Coarctation
- Critical aortic stenosis
- Tricuspid atresia
- Interrupted aortic arch.

Infancy
- VSD
- Atrioventricular septal defect (AVSD)
- Large PDA
- TAPVD.

Any age
- SVT
- Myocarditis
- Cardiomyopathy.

Signs
- Breathlessness
- Poor feeding
- Sweating
- Recurrent chest infections.

Symptoms
- Failure to thrive
- Tachypnoea
- Tachycardia
- Cardiomegaly
- Murmur/gallop rhythm
- Hepatomegaly
- Cool peripheries.

RARER PRESENTATIONS

Hypertension
Commonest causes are:

- cardiac – coarctation
- renal – reflux nephropathy secondary to urinary tract infection (UTI)
- catecholamine excess – neuroblastoma, phaeochromocytoma.

'Funny turns'

Cardiac arrhythmias

Presenting complaint
- Syncope – pallor
- Fits – blue.
  Causes
- Supraventricular tachycardia (SVT)
- Prolonged PR interval – Lown–Ganong–Levene
- Prolonged QT syndrome
  — Romano Ward (autosomal dominant (AD))
  — Jervel–Lange–Nelson (autosomal recessive (AR) + deafness)

Cerebral events

Presenting complaint
- Fit
- Transient ischaemic attack (TIA)
- Stroke.
  Causes
- Emboli – right-to-left shunt
- Thrombosis – polycythaemia
- Cerebral abscess.

Cyanotic spells
- Fallot's – infundibular spasm: 'spelling'.

Recurrent chest infections
Increased pulmonary blood flow/congestion.

- ASD
- VSD
- TAPVD.

Coincidental finding
- ECG – long QT interval
- Chest X-ray – cardiomegaly.

Subacute bacterial endocarditis

This is a very rare presentation.

COMMON LONG CASES

- Congenital heart disease
- Multisystem disorders.

CONGENITAL HEART DISEASE (CHD)

Certain congenital disorders are associated with heart disease.

Chromosomal abnormalities

- Down's syndrome (trisomy 21) – AVSD (30%), VSD, ASD
- Turner's syndrome (XO) – coarctation, aortic stenosis
- Cri-du-chat syndrome (5p–) – VSD
- Williams syndrome (microdeletion chr. 7) – supravalvular aortic stenosis, peripheral pulmonary stenosis
- Noonan's syndrome (AD, chr. 12) – pulmonary stenosis.

Intrauterine infection

- Rubella (esp. first trimester) – PDA, septal defects, peripheral pulmonary valve stenosis.

Maternal diseases

- Diabetes – increased incidence of all CHD, especially septal hypertrophy
- Systemic lupus erythematosus – congenital heart block.

Drugs in pregnancy

- Anticonvulsants – AS, PS, coarctation
- Excess alcohol – septal defects.

MULTISYSTEM DISORDERS

Some inherited causes of heart disease presenting in older children are listed below:

- Familial hypercholesterolaemia (AD) – hypertension, atherosclerosis, tendon xanthoma, corneal arcus
- Pompé's disease (type II glycogen storage disease, AD) – cardiomyopathy in infant/toddler
- Mucopolysaccharidoses (AR/X-linked) – storage material in valves may cause stenosis or regurgitation
- Marfan's syndrome (AD) – aortic regurgitation, mitral valve prolapse
- Ehlers–Danlos syndrome (AD) – aortic dissection
- Friedreich's ataxia (AR) – cardiomyopathy.

HISTORY (IMPORTANT POINTS)

Age of presentation

- Was CHD diagnosed antenatally?
- Congenital is more common than acquired

- Common associations with heart disease shown above
- 8% of CHD is associated with major chromosomal anomalies
- 10–15% is associated with non-cardiac anomalies
- If associated with a metabolic disorder, it will generally be picked up as part of routine screening once the underlying diagnosis is made. The child will usually have presented with other features of the underlying disorder.

How did it present?
- Symptomatic versus asymptomatic (see above).

Current symptoms
- Chronic limitation of exercise tolerance – quantify this
- How much school is missed?
- Headaches, 'funny turns', frequent chest infections, 'spelling'.

Family history
- Conditions associated with CHD
- Sudden/unexpected death at a young age
  — hypertrophic obstructive cardiomyopathy
  — arrythmias
  — hypercholesterolaemia.

Treatment so far
- Cardiac catheterizations or surgery
- Admission for drug therapy (suggesting previous heart failure)
- Current medications?

Immunizations up to date?
- *No vaccine is contraindicated* in CHD per se
- Measles can be particularly serious in CHD.

EXAMINATION

This is as outlined above. *Don't forget to*:

- plot height and weight on growth chart
- measure blood pressure (upper right arm, and lower limb if there is coarctation)
- comment on dental caries.

INVESTIGATIONS

You must be able to discuss the logical sequence of investigations in a child with suspected heart disease.

Arterial blood gases (ABGs)
- Essential to confirm central cyanosis
- 'Hyperoxic/nitrogen washout' test – ABG is sampled from right radial artery to confirm central cyanosis; the child is then exposed to 100% oxygen for 10 minutes and the blood gas repeated (see Table 3.5).

Table 3.5 Cyanosis

Cause	Hyperoxic test
Lung disease (unless very severe)	P_aO_2 >15 kPa
Cardiac – transposition of the great arteries (TGA), truncus arteriosus (TA), pulmonary atresia (PA), large right-to-left shunt	P_aO_2 same
Common mixing (truncus arteriosus)	modest rise in P_aO_2

Chest X-ray
- Heart – size, shape, situs
- Valves – calcified/prosthetic
- Lungs – pulmonary oligaemia/plethora/vasculature
- Bony structures – rib notching (collaterals in coarctation).

Electrocardiogram
- Axis
- Conduction abnormalities
- P-wave abnormalities
- Ventricular hypertrophy.

Echocardiogram
- Detects most cyanotic conditions in the newborn
- Very useful for acyanotic conditions (septal defects, duct or valvular disease), particularly if accompanied by Doppler measurements of flow velocity.

Cardiac catheterization
- To measure pressure gradient across stenosed valve or outflow tract obstruction
- To quantify accurately the size of the shunt
- To determine the exact anatomy of complex lesions when surgery is considered
- For intervention by dilatation of valvular stenosis or coarctation.

TREATMENT

You would be expected to know how to manage the following.

THE BLUE BABY

- Oxygen – useless unless it has been demonstrated to improve P_aO_2.
- Prostaglandin
    — Commenced if condition is 'duct-dependent', e.g. in:
        — right ventricular outflow tract obstruction
        — transposition of the great arteries (TGA)
        — left ventricular outflow tract obstruction

— Beware of side-effects:
  — hypotension
  — apnoea
  — fever
  — flushing
  — convulsions
- Correct acidosis
- Keep warm
- Prevent hypoglycaemia.

HEART FAILURE

Drugs
- Only if the child is symptomatic
- Diuretics – thiazide or loop diuretics are often used in combination with potassium-sparing to avoid the need for unpalatable potassium supplements
- ACE inhibitors – often used in conjunction with diuretics
- Digoxin – still widely prescribed although there is little evidence to support its use
- Dopamine – may be required if the child is hypotensive.

Feeding
- Passage of a nasogastric tube will reduce the work of breathing
- High-calorie feeds should be used with diuretics rather than fluid restriction as these babies often have high metabolic rates.

Monitoring
- Daily weights
- Assessment of liver size.

Ventilation
May be required for severe heart failure and for apnoea secondary to prostaglandins.

Surgery
Depends on the age of the child, but essentially there are two main reasons for performing surgery in the first year of life:

- severe heart failure with failure to thrive
- pulmonary hypertension with the potential to progress to pulmonary vascular disease.

ARRHYTHMIAS

Supraventricular tachycardia (SVT)
- The most common arrythmia in childhood
- Less than 25% have an underlying defect – commonly Wolff–Parkinson–White syndrome or Ebstein's anomaly
- If failure is evident, the arrythmia has been present for some time and treatment is urgent.

Treatment

- *Ventilation* – oxygen via mask or positive pressure
- *Circulatory support* – correction of acidosis
- *Vagal stimulation* – eyeball pressure, carotid sinus massage, submersion into ice-cold water should be tried although rarely successful in a very sick child; caution is required not to induce asystole, and thus it must always be done with a monitor attached
- *Adenosine* – this works by causing transient block of the AV node and may be of diagnostic and therapeutic benefit:
  - **diagnostic value:** if the dysrhythmia is atrial in origin, transient blockade of the AV node will slow the ventricular response to atrial tachycardia, atrial flutter and atrial fibrillation, which can then be diagnosed on the monitor. But use with caution, as there may be an accessory pathway in patients with atrial flutter or fibrillation and adenosine may increase conduction down anomalous pathways
  - **therapeutic value:** if the dysrhythmia is either AV nodal re-entry tachycardia or AV re-entry tachycardia, then adenosine may terminate the abnormal rhythm
  - **caution:** adenosine should NOT be used if the patient is on dipyrimadole, an anti-platelet drug, as dipyridamole will prolong the half-life of adenosine
- *Electrocardioversion with DC shock* – use in a severely ill child when the above has failed
- *Maintenance therapy* – digoxin or flecainide are effective.

ANTIBIOTIC PROPHYLAXIS OF ENDOCARDITIS

Prevention of endocarditis is necessary in patients with a heart-valve lesion, septal defect, patent ductus or prosthetic valve who are undergoing the following procedures:

- dental procedures, including local, general or no anaesthetic
- upper respiratory tract procedures
- genitourinary procedures
- gastrointestinal procedures
- (obstetric/gynaecological procedures).

A detailed description of antibacterial prophylaxis is given in the *British National Formulary*.

MANAGEMENT OF CONGENITAL HEART DISEASE

You need to be able to discuss the merits of medical versus surgical therapy and to be aware of current areas of debate, such as:

- How to manage VSD and when to close with surgery
- Management of ASD
- Medical or surgical treatment of PDA in the premature infant
- Management of TGA – anatomical correction versus balloon septostomy and Mustard procedure

- Total correction versus systemic to pulmonary shunt in Fallot's
- Correction of AV canal defects, especially in children with Down's syndrome.

COMMON CARDIOLOGY SHORT CASES

There is a plethora of complex congenital heart conditions but only nine common lesions, which can be categorized into acyanotic and cyanotic groups.

ACYANOTIC

Three 'holes' (left-to-right shunt)

- Ventricular septal defect (VSD)
- Atrial septal defect (ASD)
- Patent ductus arteriosus (PDA).

Three 'blocked pipes' (obstruction to flow)
- Pulmonary stenosis (PS)
- Coarctation of aorta
- Aortic stenosis (AS).

This group represents two-thirds of cases and the conditions are termed simple. The first three cases – left-to-right shunts – can lead to Eisenmenger's syndrome (pulmonary hypertension and reversal of the shunt, with consequent cyanosis). Any of the six can occur in combination but they usually occur in isolation, hence the term 'simple.'

CYANOTIC

Three 'blue babies'

- Transposition of the great arteries (TGA)
- Tetralogy of Fallot (TOF)
- Pulmonary atresia.

These account for the remaining one-third of the cases and the conditions are often complex lesions. By definition, there is a significant right-to-left shunt, or separate pulmonary and systemic circulation (transposition), but this is often complicated by other anomalies.

The algorithm for clinical examination and diagnosis (Fig. 3.8) may be helpful for the short cases as a guide to diagnosing the underlying heart disease. If you recognise the child as having an obvious syndrome then try to think of the likely underlying cardiac lesions and concentrate on the signs associated with that lesion during your examination.

Case histories of the common short cases can be found in more detail in *Paediatric Short Cases for Postgraduate Examinations* by A Thomson, H Wallace and T Stephenson (Churchill Livingstone, Edinburgh, 2003).

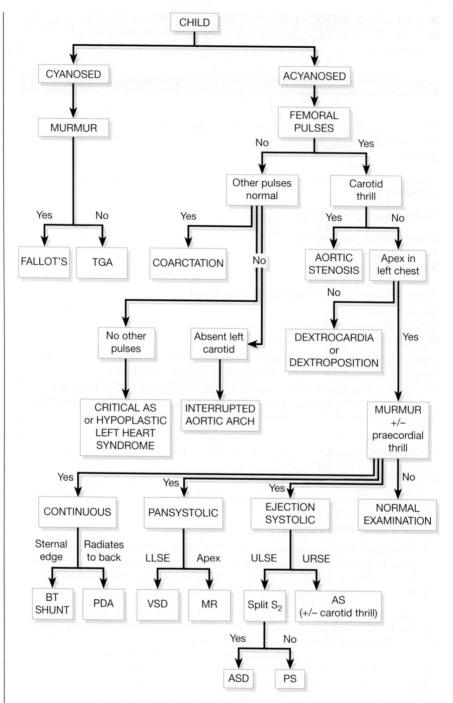

Fig 3.8 Algorithm for clinical examination.

The cardiovascular system

INSPECTION
Expose child appropriately and ideally position at 45°

Whole child
General health, nutritional status, dysmorphic features, sweating

Hands
Clubbing, peripheral cyanosis, xanthomas, splinter haemorrhages, absent thumbs, absent radii, abnormal palmar creases

Face
Plethoric, conjunctival injection, pallor, central cyanosis, teeth (conjunctival injection + gum hypertrophy = chronic cyanosis)

Chest
Respiratory rate, scars (thoracotomy = operations outside heart, sternotomy = intracardiac), symmetry – look from the side, deformity – Harrison's sulci, visible pulsation

PALPATION

Pulses
Both brachial and femoral (can do at the end), rate (count for 6 seconds then multiply by 10), quality, rhythm

BP
'I would like to measure the blood pressure at the end'

Apex
Locate apex beat (most lateral and inferior impulse) and count ribs to check position, normally fourth intercostal space in midclavicular line, nature of impulse; sustained in AS, forceful in LVH

Praecordium
Thrills or heaves, palpable P_2 in pulmonary hypertension
Suprasternal notch: thrill = aortic stenosis

AUSCULTATION

Heart sounds
- Loud S1: ASD, prosthetic valve,
- Loud S2: increased pulmonary blood flow (PDA, ASD, VSD), pulmonary hypertension
- Split S2: fixed split (ASD), wide split (ASD, PS, RBBB), reversed split (AS, LBBB)
- Single S2: tetralogy of Fallot, PS
- Extra HS: ejection click (AS/PS), mitral valve prolapse

Murmurs
Grade, timing, character, quality, position of maximum intensity, radiation (see later)

Back
Listen for murmurs and inspiratory crackles if in failure

ANYTHING ELSE?
Blood pressure
Femoral pulses
Feel for hepatomegaly
Plot height and weight on a growth chart appropriate for the patient's age and sex

INVESTIGATIONS
Saturation monitor, ABG, ECG, CXR, ECHO, cardiac catheterization

The respiratory system

4

When examining this system, the emphasis differs depending on the age of the child. The younger the child, the more important is the phase of inspection, the more difficult are palpation and percussion and the less informative is auscultation.

INSPECTION

NEONATES/INFANTS

When examining a neonate or an infant, observation provides 90% of the information. Make a point of observing. Listen as well as look.

Do not undress an infant until you know the following:

- respiratory rate
- colour
- nasal flaring, using accessory muscles
- stridor (inspiration > expiration), wheeze (expiration > inspiration).

GENERAL

- General health e.g. nutritional status, failure to thrive
- Dysmorphic features.
- Extras – oxygen supplementation, saturation monitors, sputum pots, peak flow meters.

HANDS

Clubbing (usually cystic fibrosis in exams but may be due to other lung conditions causing chronic infection or hypoxia).

FACE

Cyanosis (respiratory failure); traumatic petechiae on the eyelids, face and neck may be seen following severe paroxysms of coughing.

NECK

Tracheal tug, swellings, lymph nodes, cystic hygroma, thyroid.

CHEST

Undress the top half of the child completely, down to the waist, except in the case of an adolescent girl.

Shape

- Asymmetry
  - diminution on one side
  - lung collapse, fibrosis or spinal deformity
- Deformity
  - check spine for scoliosis or kyphosis
  - ask older children to touch toes to determine whether postural
- Pectus excavatum – sunken sternum
- Pectus carinatum – prominent sternum (pigeon chest)
- Hyperinflation
  - barrel chest: increased AP diameter
  - chronic asthma, emphysema, CF
- Harrison's sulcus
  - retracted costal cartilages; flaring lower ribs
  - chronic airways obstruction
  - left-to-right cardiac shunt
- Rachitic rosary
  - swelling of costochondral junctions
  - rickets
- Absent clavicles – cleidocranial dysostosis
- Absent pectoralis – Poland's syndrome
- Movement
  - compare both sides
  - full expiration, followed by inspiration.

Recession

- Intercostal – airways obstruction or decreased lung compliance
- Subcostal – airways obstruction or decreased lung compliance.

Scars

- Sternotomy – usually cardiac surgery
- Left thoracotomy
  - repair coarctation
  - Blalock–Taussig (BT) shunt
  - lobectomy
- Right thoracotomy
  - oesophageal surgery
  - BT shunt
  - lobectomy
- Previous chest drains.

Rate (Table 4.1)

Count the rate for a minimum of 10 seconds by watching the chest or abdomen move. Watch for any signs of increased work of breathing, such as:

- nasal flaring
- grunting on expiration – raised positive end-expiratory pressure
- using accessory muscles – especially sternocleidomastoids
- intercostal indrawing – chest wall recession
- use of abdominal muscles for expiration
- see-saw chest and abdominal movement – abdomen moves out with forceful diaphragm contraction and chest sucked in; recesses during forced inspiration
- difficulty feeding/speaking.

Table 4.1 Respiratory rate in children

Age	Normal range (breaths/min)	Tachypnoea (breaths/min)
Neonate	30–60	>60
Infant	20–40	>50
1–3 years	20–30	>40
4–10 years	15–25	>35
>10 years	15–20	>30

PALPATION

Be guided by the age of the child.

YOUNG CHILD/INFANT

- Palpation and percussion are not part of the routine, except:
  - to assess the degree of hyperinflation
  - to detect upper border of the liver
  - to confirm signs of consolidation, collapse or effusion.
- A young child's chest shape is circular and breathing is abdominal and diaphragmatic, thus chest expansion is pointless.
- Respiratory distress is indicated by use of accessory muscles, and dyspnoea is reflected by increased abdominal movements.
- Over-inflation is most evident in the upper half of the chest (e.g. in bronchiolitis or chronic lung disease).

OLDER CHILD

Mediastinum position (Table 4.2)
- Feel the trachea – single finger in the midline
- Localize apex beat.

Chest expansion
Place your hands on the chest with your fingers grasping the sides of the chest in such a way that the outstretched thumbs approximate at the tips,

Table 4.2 Mediastinal position

Apex and trachea Pushed away	Pulled towards	Only trachea shifted	Only apex shifted
Pleural effusion (may be no shift if underlying lung collapse)	Collapse	Upper lobe pathology	Pectus excavatum
Pneumothorax	Fibrosis		Scoliosis Dextrocardia (think Kartagener's) Cardiomegaly (think cor pulmonale)

Table 4.3 Tactile vocal fremitus

Vibrations	Pathology on that side
Increased	Consolidation
Decreased	Collapse Pleural thickening
Absent	Pleural effusion

without touching the chest, to allow free movement in expansion. To measure maximum chest expansion, ask the child to breathe all the way out, then to take a big breath in. Make sure your fingers remain tightly (but not painfully) applied to the chest wall so that the thumbs act as 'calipers'. Anteriorly, the thumbs should be placed at the level of the nipples, while posteriorly, the thumbs should be at T10 level. Chest expansion can be measured in an older child and should be at least 4 cm. Diminution of movement on one side indicates pathology on that side. Both hyperinflation and restrictive lung disease can reduce expansion symmetrically, and formal pulmonary function testing provides more reliable information.

Tactile vocal fremitus (Table 4.3)

This provides exactly the same information as vocal resonance – do not do both. We recommend doing vocal resonance as pathology is more easily detected. To test tactile vocal fremitus, place the palm of the hand on either side of the upper chest and ask the child to say '99'. Most children will happily engage in the game. Compare right and left, anteriorly and posteriorly.

PERCUSSION (Table 4.4)

- Always tell the child what you are going to do. To avoid scaring him with a resounding blow to the chest, say: 'I am going to make you sound like a drum.'
- Percuss with the middle finger of the right hand at right angles to the middle phalanx of the left hand laid flat on the chest, with the movement coming from the wrist. The commonest mistake is not pressing hard enough with the left hand, so that a muffled percussion note results.

Table 4.4 Percussion note

Note	Pathology
Resonant	Normal lung
Hyperresonant	Pneumothorax Emphysema
Dull	Consolidation Collapse Pleural thickening Fibrosis
Stony dull	Pleural effusion

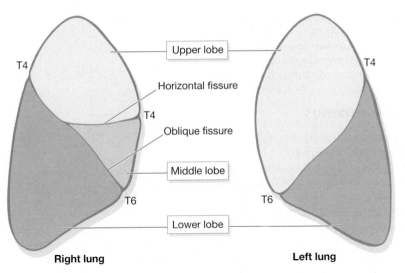

Right lung   Left lung

Fig. 4.1 Surface anatomy in relation to lung lobes.

- Be aware of the surface anatomy in relation to lung lobes (Fig. 4.1).
- Tap twice at each of the sites shown in Figure 4.2.
- Always compare right with left.
- Don't forget to percuss the upper border of the liver (sixth intercostal space anteriorly).
- Continue with auscultation on the front of the chest before percussing the back.

AUSCULTATION

- Explain to the child that you are going to listen to his chest. Do not ask.
- Demonstrate on teddy if the child is reluctant.
- Do not give up if the child is upset; listen to inspiratory breaths, between cries if necessary.
- You must use a paediatric stethoscope, not an adult or a neonatal one.
- The bell or diaphragm of the stethoscope can be used for auscultation.

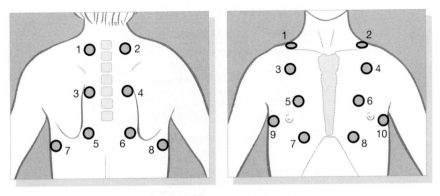

Fig. 4.2 Sites for percussion.

- Listen over the same area as for percussion, for two breaths.
- Ask yourself three questions:
  — Are the breath sounds normal?
  — Are there added sounds?
  — Are these in inspiration, expiration or both?

BREATH SOUNDS

Normal (vesicular) (Fig. 4.3)
- Low-pitched rustle
- Increase in intensity in inspiration
- Fades quickly in first third of expiration.

Abnormal breath sounds (Table 4.5)
Breath sounds can be abnormal in three ways.

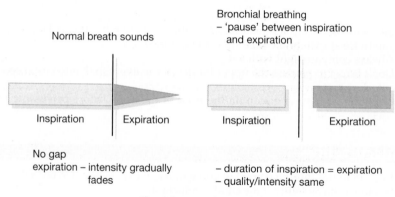

Fig. 4.3 Breath sounds.

Table 4.5 Abnormal breath sounds	
Breath sounds	**Pathology**
Diminished or absent	Collapse
	Pleural effusion
	Pneumothorax
	Pleural thickening
	Emphysema
	Obstruction, e.g. tumour
Bronchial	Consolidation
	Fibrosis
Prolonged expiration	Asthma
	Emphysema

Diminished or absent
- No airflow or conduction attenuated by air or fluid.

Bronchial (Fig. 4.3)
- Patent bronchi, but solid alveoli
- Inspiration and expiration both give a harsh blowing sound
- Duration of inspiration is equal to that of expiration
- Pause between inspiration and expiration
- Breath sounds are harsh and can be simulated by listening over the trachea during breathing.

Prolonged expiration
- In asthma or emphysema
- To prevent closure of alveoli.

Added sounds

Conducted upper airway sounds   These sounds make examination of young children very difficult and are the cause of most false-positive findings. Most infants 'gurgle' and many toddlers are 'snotty'. Remember that serious bacterial infections tend to localize (one ear, one joint, one lung lobe), whereas viral upper respiratory tract infections have wider effects (red eyes, runny nose, red throat, skin rash, myalgia, etc.). These sounds are heard without a stethoscope and will remain as background noise when auscultating. A useful ploy is to place the stethoscope on the side of the neck after listening to the chest. If coarse, variable crackles heard in the chest are obviously louder over the neck, they are certainly conducted upper airways sounds.

Wheezes
- High-pitched musical noises due to partial obstruction or narrowing of bronchi or bronchioles
- Maximal on expiration, which is usually prolonged (the positive intrapleural pressure accompanying forced expiration further reduces the lumen of intrathoracic airways)
- Can occur in inspiration if obstruction is severe; tends to be lower-pitched.
  Common causes
- Asthma (only one likely in the exam)
- Bronchiolitis (accompanied by crepitations).
  Less common (unilateral) causes
- Foreign body or other cause of fixed localized (large) airway narrowing, e.g. stenosis.

Crackles   These are non-musical sounds, generally heard during inspiration:

- Fine, high-pitched at the bases, alveolar level
  — pulmonary oedema
  — fibrosing alveolitis (especially at the end of inspiration)
- Coarse, variable pitch, bubbly secretions in bronchioles
  — pneumonia
  — bronchiectasis.

The second condition in each of the above cases is rarer but more likely in the exam. **NB.** Check whether the crackles clear after coughing.

Pleural sounds

Pleural rub
- Leathery sound caused by movement of visceral pleura over parietal pleura, when the surfaces are roughened as by fibrinous exudate (pleurisy) – uncommon in children.

Pneumothorax click
- Rhythmical sound, synchronous with cardiac systole
- Heard with or without a stethoscope
- Caused by shallow left pneumothorax between the two layers overlying the heart.

VOCAL RESONANCE

Do not do this if you have already assessed for tactile vocal fremitus.
NB. Alterations of breath sounds and vocal resonance depend on the same criteria and alter together.

- Ask the child to say '99' whilst listening over the same areas as during auscultation. The findings are the same as for tactile vocal fremitus, but the sounds are louder over areas of consolidation.
- At the surface of an effusion, the words '99' sound like a bleating goat (*aegophony*). In some cases the sounds can be transmitted clearly when whispering, without voice distortion, known as *whispering pectoriloquy.*
- Having completed examination of the front of the chest, ask the child to sit forward and repeat the sequence on the back. Don't forget to examine for lymphadenopathy if you have not already done so.

Table 4.6 presents a summary of the physical signs that manifest in respiratory diseases.

COMMON LONG CASES

- Chronic asthma
- Cystic fibrosis
- Chronic lung disease.

It is important that you are prepared for these long cases, which are commonly encountered in the exam. You must be well rehearsed in history-taking and examination appropriate to each of the conditions. Furthermore, you will need to know the appropriate investigations and management and be able to discuss current topical issues.

CHRONIC ASTHMA

Asthma can be defined as 'recurrent reversible small airways obstruction'.

HISTORY

Evidence
What is the evidence from the parents that the child has asthma?

- Documented reversibility of wheeze with bronchodilators
- Persistent cough and admissions with vague 'chestiness'

Table 4.6 Physical signs in respiratory diseases

	Chest movement	Mediastinal shift	Percussion note	Vocal resonance	Breath sounds
Pleural effusion	Decreased	To opposite side	Stony dull	Absent	Absent +/- bronchial sounds above fluid level
Consolidation	Decreased	None	Dull	Increased + whispering pectoriloquy	Bronchial +/- crackles
Collapse	Decreased	To same side	Dull	Decreased	Decreased
Fibrosis	Decreased	To same side	Dull	Increased	Bronchial +/- crackles
Pneumothorax	Decreased	To opposite side	Resonant	Decreased	Decreased

- Chonic nocturnal cough
- Shortness of breath on exercise without wheeze.

Age of onset
Is there any relevant prior respiratory illness, e.g. respiratory distress syndrome, bronchiolitis?

Precipitants
- Upper respiratory tract infections
- Exercise and emotion
- House dust mite
- Grass pollen
- Seasonal variation (spring and autumn peaks)
- Animal dander (ask about pets)
- Parental cigarette smoking, especially maternal smoking (both ante- and postnatal)
- Damp housing (mouldy)
- Particular environmental settings, e.g. visits to the country.

Measures taken to reduce exposure to house dust
- Synthetic bedclothes and pillows
- 'Hypoallergenic' cover for the mattress/pillow/duvet
- Nylon carpet in the child's bedroom
- Frequent vacuum cleaning of the bedroom/damp dusting.

These are clearly expensive and inconvenient changes for most families to make and the rewards may be limited. Compliance with these measures, therefore, suggests asthma which has been difficult to control.

Severity and chronicity of symptoms
- How frequent are the symptoms?
- How is it affecting the child's life?
- Can he/she keep up with peers at school?
- How many days are missed per school term?
- How often is sleep disturbed?
- How often are the 'reliever' inhalers used per month?
- Courses of oral steroids?

Family history of asthma or atopy
Is there such a family history, especially in the mother and other first-degree relatives?

Passive smoking
Do any family members smoke cigarettes?

Treatment
- What is the current treatment, and what are the dose and frequency?
- What inhaler devices have been used?
- What previous treatments have been tried and have failed?
- Are home nebulizers used for difficult asthma?

Peak flow diary

This may show diurnal variation and morning dips, suggesting continuing airway lability.

PATTERN

You should now have an understanding of the pattern of asthma that the child has:

- acute and infrequent (if any) spells when asymptomatic
- episodic, frequent attacks, with complete resolution in between attacks.
- chronic with persistence of symptoms between attacks.

EXAMINATION

- Failure to thrive – poorly controlled asthma
- 'Extras' – oxygen, nebulizers, inhalers around the bed
- Atopy? – eczema, conjunctivitis, rhinitis or a crease on the nose from constant rubbing with the palm of the hand ('hay fever salute'). A Morgan–Dennie fold is a double fold under the eye in eczematous or allergic children
- Examine the nose with an auriscope and large speculum. Atopic mucosa is pale and oedematous with watery mucus present
- Cushinoid appearance? Measure blood pressure
- Signs of chronic asthma:
  — Harrison's sulcus
  — hyperinflation
  — persistent recession and wheeze despite bronchodilators
- Record pulse, pulsus paradoxus, respiratory rate and temperature, as the child may have come into hospital with an acute exacerbation
- Check the child's inhaler technique
- Measure the peak expiratory flow rate (PEFR):

Average PEFR (L/min) = (5 × height in cm) − 400

The third centile peak flow for a given height is 50 L/min less than the average. To ensure the test is done properly the child must be > 5 years old.

INVESTIGATIONS

Asthma is a clinical diagnosis and investigations should be kept to a minimum.

Chest X-ray
- At first presentation – to exclude a foreign body and provide a baseline
- To exclude pneumothorax, if clinically suspected
- Patchy collapse/consolidation is common during an acute attack due to airways obstruction and antibiotics should be used on clinical grounds rather than on X-ray appearances.

Arterial blood gases
- Only useful in acute situations
- Capillary blood gases from a warm extremity will give reliable CO_2 and pH data.

Lung function tests
- Serial peak flow measurements can be useful
- Outpatient therapy is generally titrated against clinical performance
- It can be helpful to demonstrate that obstruction is not reversible (e.g. obliterative bronchiolitis) or that there is coexistent restrictive lung disease (e.g. cystic fibrosis or fibrosing alveolitis)
- Spirometry may be a more sensitive test than peak expiratory flow for assessing airway obstruction
- Histamine challenge may be beneficial for assessment of degree of bronchial hyperactivity.

Skin tests
- Most specific allergens (e.g. cats, horse, grass) will be obvious from the history
- There is a poor correlation between skin and bronchial reactivity
- Many false positives and a remote possibility of anaphylaxis
- The only treatment is allergen avoidance.

MANAGEMENT

Asthma is a common long case, and as most candidates have plenty of practical experience, it is difficult to excel. To do well you must be familiar with commonly discussed topics and be aware of the controversial issues in the management of asthma.

Acute exacerbation
Know the 'danger signs' (Table 4.7). Figure 4.4 provides an algorithm for the management of acute exacerbation of asthma. You must know the detailed management of acute severe asthma, including interpretation of blood gases and indications for referral to intensive care, for discussion in the long case and oral examination.

Long-term management
- Establish the pattern of asthma
- Prescribe appropriate drugs (see below)
- Patient/parent education:
  — drugs to be used and when
  — understanding of roles of 'relievers and preventers'
  — inhaler technique
  — management of acute exacerbation

Table 4.7 The 'danger signs'	
Severe	**Life-threatening**
Too breathless to feed or speak	Restlessness (hypoxia)
Respiratory rate >50/min	Drowsiness (hypercapnia)
Pulse >140/min	Peak flow <33% of predicted or best
Peak flow <50% predicted or best	Exhaustion
Pulsus paradoxus >15 mmHg	Silent chest
	Cyanosis

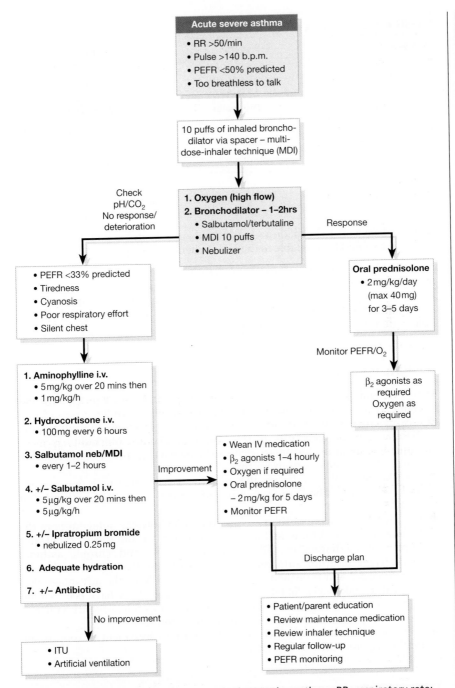

Fig. 4.4 Management of acute severe/life-threatening asthma. RR, respiratory rate; b.p.m., beats per minute; PEFR, peak expiratory flow rate; i.v., intravenous; ITU, intensive care unit; neb, nebulizer.

Clinical paediatrics for postgraduate exams

Table 4.8 Choosing the correct inhaler

<4 years	4–9 years	>9 years
	Dry powder Turbohaler Acuhaler Disc-haler	Dry powder Turbohaler Acuhaler Disc-haler
Metered dose inhaler – via spacer and mask	Metered dose inhaler – via spacer	Metered dose inhaler
Nebulizer	Nebulizer	Nebulizer

- School teachers to be made aware of the diagnosis and to know that the inhaler should be available to the child when necessary.

You must be familiar with the current *British Thoracic Guidelines* for the stepwise approach to ensuring good control and also have an understanding of the method of action of these drugs (Fig. 4.5). It is essential that you are familiar with the various delivery systems and are able to demonstrate their use if requested (Table 4.8).

TOPICAL ISSUES

- Use of antibiotics in exacerbations of asthma – viral infections are the commonest precipitants in younger children, especially in winter.
- Despite increased awareness and improved treatment, mortality from asthma has changed little in the last two decades. Morbidity is more difficult to quantify. Incidence seems to be increasing. You should be able to discuss the possible reasons for this.
- You should be able to discuss the side-effects associated with oral steroids and the debates about the potential side-effects associated with inhaled steroids.
- You should be aware of the possible role of leukotriene antagonists in the management of chronic asthma. Leukotrienes are the most potent and important mediators of inflammation in acute and chronic asthma. Leukotriene-receptor antagonists, such as Montelukast, have both anti-inflammatory and bronchodilator properties and have the advantage that they can be taken as a tablet once or twice per day. They have been shown to be effective in adults over a wide spectrum of asthma severity, either as monotherapy or in combination with inhaled steroids.
- You should consider whether the child's current treatment is appropriate for the apparent asthma severity.

CYSTIC FIBROSIS (CF)

This is an autosomally inherited, fatal, multisystem disorder. The carrier frequency is 1:20–25, giving an incidence of 1:2000 and correlating with a prevalence of approximately 7000 patients with CF in the UK. As 50–80% of children survive to adult life, it is a disorder commonly seen in the exam. There are now as many adults as children with CF in the UK.

Step 1	Step 2	Step 3	Step 4	Step down
	Cromoglicate or inhaled steroids	Inhaled steroid + long-acting β_2 agonist (Salmeterol) and/or leukotriene receptor antagonist (Montelukast)	Inhaled steroid + long-acting β_2 agonist (Salmeterol) and/or leukotriene receptor antagonist (Montelukast) + alternate day prednisolone	Step down treatment when good control achieved
β_2 bronchodilator	β_2 bronchodilator	β_2 bronchodilator	β_2 bronchodilator	β_2 bronchodilator

Fig. 4.5 Pharmacological management of chronic asthma.

HISTORY

Age of onset and symptoms at presentation

- CF is mostly diagnosed in infants and toddlers who present with either or both of the following:
  - recurrent cough or chest infections (50%)
  - failure to thrive despite a good intake (30%); over 90% of children with diagnosed CF have malabsorption and steatorrhoea due to pancreatic exocrine enzyme insufficiency.
- 10% present in the neonatal period with meconium ileus, a misnomer as there is mechanical obstruction due to inspissated meconium rather than ileus. There is often an associated micro-colon. Ask the parent if he or she can remember at what age meconium was first passed – 48 hours or more would be noteworthy. Recently, delay in passing meconium has been shown to be related to the effect of the CF modifier gene on chromosome 19.
- Toddlers rarely present with rectal prolapse.
- A few cases are not diagnosed until school age or later.
- Some cases are detected by screening in a family with an index case.

Ongoing symptoms

- Frequency of chest infections requiring oral/intravenous antibiotics
- Amount of school missed
- Exercise tolerance
- Frequency of cough
- Amount of sputum produced
- Persistent abnormalities of bowel habit or stools despite treatment
- Recurrent episodes of abdominal pain due to meconium ileus equivalent (now called distal intestinal obstruction syndrome).

Complications

Respiratory

- Sinusitis, often associated with recurrent nasal polyps
- Known bacterial infection – *Staphylococcus aureus, Haemophilus influenzae, Pseudomonas aeruginosa* or *Burkholderia cepacia*, atypical mycobacteria
- Bronchial hyperreactivity with wheeze and evidence of reversible airway obstruction
- Allergic bronchopulmonary aspergillosis
- Minor haemoptysis is common – usually related to respiratory infection
- Major haemoptysis, in older children and adults, is rare and may require angiography and bronchial artery embolization
- Progressive decline in lung function leading to respiratory failure and the development of cor pulmonale.

GI/endocrine

- There is an increased incidence of coeliac disease and Crohn's disease
- Growth failure and delayed puberty have traditionally been thought to correlate better with the severity of respiratory disease. However, it has been shown that improvement in nutrition itself results in less severe respiratory disease and improved growth
- Diabetes mellitus – prevalence increases with age
- Liver cirrhosis +/– portal hypertension (prevalence does not increase with age)

- A detailed nutritional history is essential as inadequate dietary intake compounds the energy deficiency resulting from malabsorption and increased work of breathing.

Family history
- Other siblings may be affected
- Has the family had counselling about the risk associated with subsequent pregnancies?

Treatment regimens
- Postural drainage and physiotherapy regimens
- Prophylactic antibiotics – inhaled or oral
- Current antibiotics for intercurrent infection
- Inhaled bronchodilators or steroids
- Mucolytics – DNAse
- Pancreatic supplements
- Antacids or proton pump inhibitors
- Vitamin supplements (fat-soluble)
- Overnight nutritional support (past and present) – gastric tube feeding overnight, parenteral nutrition, nutritional supplements orally.

Immunizations
- Obtain a detailed history of past immunizations – ask specifically if the child has been immunized against pertussis and measles, both of which can be particularly nasty in CF patients.
- Does the child routinely receive influenza vaccine each autumn?

Psychological/psychosocial impact
- Teenage patients have particular problems with time missed from school, short stature and delayed puberty resulting in poor body image.
- What has been the effect on the child's school performance?
- What is the child's and family's understanding of the reason behind all the treatments given?
- What has been the impact on the rest of the family of a child with a chronic, debilitating, fatal disease requiring frequent hospital attendances and admissions?
- What is the availability of financial support to the family, e.g. Disability Living Allowance, Mobility Allowance, Invalid Allowance?

EXAMINATION

Clinical features are very variable, in terms of both the systems involved and the severity.

General
- Well or unwell?
- Nutritional status: – height and weight are essential measurements; estimate the expected weight for height and calculate the present weight as a percentage of the ideal weight
- Febrile or not?
- Extras – oxygen, pulse oximeter, sputum pots, inhalers
- Tunnelled central venous access in situ?

Respiratory
- Clubbing – occurs early in CF and is not related to the severity
- Chest shape:
  — hyperinflation with pectus carinatum
  — +/– kyphosis
  — Harrison's sulcus
- Increased respiratory effort at rest
  — tachypnoea
  — using accessory muscles for both inspiration and expiration
- Bronchiectasis is suggested by coarse crackles which do not clear with coughing
- Nasal airway – is there obstruction of either nostril due to nasal polyps?
- Cyanosis, pulmonary hypertension and cor pulmonale are late signs.

Abdomen
- Gastrostomy tube in situ
- Scars suggesting surgery for neonatal or later bowel obstruction
- Palpable liver
  — due to hyperinflated chest
  — may be enlarged (although the liver is frequently involved, there is rarely hepatomegaly)
- Splenomegaly may result from portal hypertension; if so, look for other signs of advanced cirrhosis (Ch. 5)
- Palpable masses in the right iliac fossa are most likely to be faeces, which may be adherent to the bowel wall and a cause of recurrent abdominal pain.

Pubertal staging
Puberty is often delayed in these children.

INVESTIGATIONS

Prenatal diagnosis and screening
You must be able to discuss prenatal diagnosis both in general terms (biochemical markers, genetic markers, amniocentesis versus cordocentesis versus chorionic villus biopsy, ultrasound, which population to screen, etc.) and with specific reference to CF.

Carrier screening   This is offered at some centres to mothers booking in early pregnancy. A blood or mouthwash sample is screened for the six common CF gene mutations, resulting in an 85% detection rate of CF-carrier mothers. Partners of carrier mothers are then also offered screening and prenatal diagnosis can be performed for those couples who are both found to be carriers. Termination of pregnancy would be offered if the fetus was found to be affected by CF. This screening technique may reduce the number of new babies affected by CF by up to 50%.

Neonatal screening   This is carried out in some regions using measurements of immunoreactive trypsin (IRT) on a Guthrie card sample. IRT is high in a neonate with CF. This test is sensitive but not very specific. High IRT levels combined with ΔF508 mutation analysis, which can also be carried out on a Guthrie card sample, improves the specificity of the neonatal screening.

   CF screening results in earlier diagnosis of index cases, and studies have shown that the initiation of early treatment in groups of patients diagnosed by neonatal screening gives an early nutritional advantage. No significant long-term pulmonary advantage of early diagnosis by screening has yet been shown and therefore neonatal screening has not been universally adopted. Screening also provides the possibility of genetic counselling for further pregnancies.

DIAGNOSIS

Sweat test
Although this remains the standard test for CF, some patients with uncommon mutations may have repeatedly normal sweat tests. False positives and negatives are also possible if the test is incorrectly performed by inexperienced technicians. Sweat is collected by pilocarpine iontophoresis onto filter paper (Gibson & Cook) or liquid sweat can be collected in a capillary tube (Wescor). A minimum of 100 mg of sweat must be collected. A sweat sodium of over 70 mmol/L on two occasions is diagnostic. Sweat chloride in affected patients usually exceeds sweat sodium concentration. Sweat tests in the first 6 weeks of life are unreliable.

A falsely elevated sweat test can result from:

- adrenal insufficiency
- nephrogenic diabetes insipidus
- ectodermal dysplasia
- hypothyroidism
- hypopituitarism
- glycogen storage disease type I
- fucosidosis
- HIV infection
- severe malnutrition.

Immunoreactive trypsin (IRT)
This is unreliable after the first 2 months of life.

Nasal potential difference testing
CF patients have an increased potential difference across (nasal respiratory) epithelium – 45 versus 15 mV in normal children. This technique is only used as a research tool at present.

Gene testing
The CF gene lies on the long arm of chromosome 7. This is a large gene of 250 kb and over 950 mutations within the CF gene have been described. The commonest CF mutation in the UK is ΔF508, accounting for approximately 78% of CF patients. This mutation, ΔF508, indicates that three base-pairs have been deleted from the CF gene resulting in the omission of one phenylalanine amino acid from the protein (the CF transmembrane conductance regulator protein) encoded by the gene. The cystic fibrosis transmembrane regulator (CFTR) is a membrane protein. This membrane protein is an energy-dependent cyclic AMP-mediated chloride ion channel. Patients with CF have either no CFTR or defective CFTR in the cell membrane of affected tissues. Different CF gene mutations produce a range of problems in CF gene transcription, CFTR production, migration of CFTR to atypical cell membrane or CFTR gene functioning. More than 300 polymorphisms not apparently related to abnormal gene/CFTR function have also been identified.

Clinical paediatrics for postgraduate exams

TREATMENT

Effective management requires a multidisciplinary approach, involving paediatricians, physiotherapists, nursing staff, dieticians, the primary care team, the child and the child's family in order to delay the progression of lung disease and to maintain adequate nutrition and growth.

Respiratory

Physiotherapy   All CF patients require regular physiotherapy at least twice daily. Postural drainage and percussion are routine for infants and young children; older children may be allowed more independence with postural drainage and special breathing techniques. Compliance may be a problem in teenagers.

Physical exercise   Regular vigorous physical exercise should be encouraged as tolerated to strengthen the muscles and prevent reaccumulation of secretions.

Prompt treatment of infections   Antibiotic therapy in CF is controversial. Most centres start oral flucloxacillin following diagnosis, e.g. in the neonatal period. Acute infections require treatment with an antibiotic appropriate for the organism's sensitivities. Vigorous attempts should be made to prevent colonization by *Pseudomonas aeruginosa* or *Burkholderia cepacia* – treatment is with ciprofloxacin orally and nebulized Colomycin/tobramycin for up to 3 months. Intravenous antibiotics, including tobramycin, are likely to be required for acute infections. Nebulized antibiotics, Colomycin and tobramycin, reduce the frequency of respiratory exacerbations in patients colonized with *Pseudomonas cepacia*.

Nebulized acetylcysteine   This has not been proven to be of significant benefit.

Mucolytics   such as dornase, a DNAse agent, are new drugs which significantly reduce sputum viscosity and increase mucociliary clearance. Short-term trials have shown a mean 5–10% improvement in lung function over a 6-month period.

Inhaled bronchodilators and steroids   β-Sympathomimetics should be used before physiotherapy if an element of reversible airways obstruction has been demonstrated (up to 30% of cases). Inhaled steroids are also frequently used for these patients (after physiotherapy).

Long-term oral steroids   These remain controversial. Their use is intended as anti-inflammatory therapy. There is no established safe dosage for long-term treatment, which has been shown to be associated with unacceptable side-effects such as diabetes, cataracts and growth suppression.

Prophylactic antibiotics   Although this is a controversial area, most centres practise this policy to prevent persistent bacterial infection with *Staphylococcus* in infancy. Long-term nebulized antibiotics are given to patients chronically colonized with *Pseudomonas aeruginosa*.

Nutrition

Chronic undernutrition is receiving increasing recognition as an adverse prognostic factor in CF as it has been shown to lead to failure to thrive and stunting of growth and inversely correlates to survival. Management centres on restoring the energy imbalance in the form of nutritional supplementation.

Pancreatic enzyme supplements   Pancreatic enzyme preparations consist of enteric-coated microspheres within a gelatin capsule and are given with all meals and snacks. The use of high-dose pancreatic enzyme supplements has been associated with reports of strictures of the terminal ileum requiring partial colectomy when used in excessive dosage. The current recommended daily dose is 10 000 units lipase/kg, although many patients may take between 10 000 and 20 000 units/day.

H_2 blockers/proton pump inhibitors   The dissolution of the microspheres and pancreatic enzyme activity is maximal at about pH 5–5.5. Absent pancreatic bicarbonate secretion and poor neutralization of stomach acid result in reduced efficacy of pancreatic enzyme supplements. H_2 blockers have not been shown significantly to improve pancreatic enzyme activity. Omeprazole, a protein pump blocker, is probably more effective.

High-calorie diet   With an energy requirement 30–40% greater than the average recommended for age and height, a high-fat, high-calorie diet is essential to maintain adequate calorie intake. Continuous overnight enteral feeding either by nasogastric tube or by gastrostomy is useful for patients who are unable to maintain weight for height >85% with improved dietary supplements and regular meals with snacks during the day. Improved weight gain can usually be achieved, and is often accompanied by increased well-being. In many clinics, at least 10% of patients will receive supplementary enteral feeding, usually overnight.

Vitamin supplements   Regular fat-soluble vitamins (ADEK) as supplements are required.

Bowel care   Meconium ileus presenting in the newborn period may respond to gastrografin/water-soluble enemas. Intestinal obstruction failing to respond to medical treatment may require laparotomy +/– ileostomy. Distal intestinal obstruction syndrome (DIOS) is characterized by palpable faecal lumps in the caecum and ascending colon. These may cause colicky abdominal pain sometimes associated with meals, leading to subacute or complete intestinal obstruction.

Monitoring for liver disease   A high percentage of older children have some degree of hepatic fibrosis, but full-blown biliary cirrhosis develops in only about 5%. This leads to portal hypertension and, although rare, children can present with oesophageal variceal bleeding.

Monitoring for diabetes mellitus   Glucose intolerance is found in up to 75% of patients with insulin-dependent diabetes occurring in 9% of 5–9 year-olds, 26% of 10–19 year-olds, 35% of 20–30 year-olds and 45% in those over 30.

Psychological counselling

This may be required for children and parents, especially when patients reach teenage years. Common problems are:

- poor body image
- delayed pubertal development
- boys are usually infertile
- girls may have reduced fertility due to increased stickiness of cervical mucus
- girls will require contraceptive advice
- pregnancy is often associated with significant maternal decline in lung function following delivery
- the death of contemporaries who attend the same clinic/ward.

Long-term 'cure'

Lung transplantation   This is the ultimate rescue therapy for CF patients in respiratory failure. The mean survival following lung or heart–lung transplantation is approximately 70% at 2 years. Quality of life is significantly enhanced but lifelong immunosuppression with ciclosporin, azathioprine and prednisolone will be required.

- CF does not affect the transplanted lungs as it is a genetic condition of the tissues and the donor organs have normal CFTR.
- Post-transplant CF patients usually experience significant weight gain despite a reduction in calorie intake.
- Finger clubbing usually regresses.

Gene therapy   A cDNA copy of messenger RNA for normal CFTR can be transfected into CF respiratory epithelial cells using either a modified adenovirus or liposome as a vector to carry the cDNA into the cell. Early clinical trials are underway to address the safety and efficacy questions. It seems likely that, if successful, the patients who will benefit most from gene therapy are those who have preserved lung function and minimal established lung damage. To date, gene therapy trials have not proved sufficiently effective at adequately correcting the cellular defect to be introduced more widely. Repeated administration of CFTR using an adenovirus vector results in progressively less effective gene transfer, probably due to the development of blocking antibodies.

CHRONIC LUNG DISEASE (BRONCHOPULMONARY DYSPLASIA)

This is the commonest serious chronic lung disease affecting infants under 1 year of age in the UK. Such children are now relatively commonly used as long cases in the Membership examination.

   A major determinant of survival in very premature neonates is difficulty with ventilation associated with lung immaturity. As respiratory support has improved, the survival of preterm infants has increased and consequently the incidence of chronic lung disease is rising and has been shown in some studies to occur in up to 50% of very low birthweight babies.

Definition Chronic lung disease of prematurity, formerly known as BPD, is a consequence of barotrauma and volume trauma resulting from artificial ventilation, oxygen toxicity and infection in the immature lungs and is defined as lung damage associated with oxygen dependency at 36 weeks post-conceptual age (i.e. gestational age at birth plus postnatal age). There is a move away from the old term of bronchopulmonary dysplasia, which was used to describe radiological appearances in the damaged lung, as a consequence of artificial ventilation, and an oxygen dependency at 28 days of life.

HISTORY

Antenatal details
● Antenatal dexamethasone – number of courses
● Timing of rupture of membranes.

Delivery
● Requirement for active resuscitation
● Evidence of aspiration syndrome?
● Surfactant.

Neonatal intensive care
● Duration – including length of time O_2 by day, O_2 by night
● Ventilation
  — conventional versus high-frequency oscillation
  — steroids
  — chest drains for pneumothoraces
● Other problems
  — patent ductus arteriosus: use of indomethacin, ligation
  — necrotizing enterocolitis
  — intraventricular haemorrhage/periventricular leucomalacia
  — retinopathy of prematurity.

Discharge
● Home oxygen – supply of oxygen concentrators/cylinders, portable oxygen
● Monitoring
  — apnoea monitors: true and false alarms
  — pulse oximetry
  — sleep studies.

Intercurrent infections
● GP call-outs/hospital admissions
● Frequency and severity of symptoms of coryza and wheeze
● Feeding difficulties
● Weight gain.

Support
● Community nurses.

Additional risk factors for sudden infant death syndrome (SIDS)
- Passive smoking
- Bottle-feeding
- Prone sleeping position
- Heating in the bedroom or excessive bedclothes.

Medication
- Inhalers – ipratropium bromide, β_2-agonists, inhaler devices
- Vitamin, calcium and phosphate supplements
- Nutritional supplements.

EXAMINATION

General
- Failure to thrive – plot length, weight and OFC on appropriate centile chart, using corrected gestational age.

Respiratory/CVS
- Oxygen therapy – nasal cannulae, oxygen cylinders, rate of oxygen delivery, monitoring equipment
- Respiratory rate, pulse, respiratory effort – may be tachypnoeic, with intercostal and subcostal recession and hyperinflation, even if well
- Scars – chest drains, lateral thoracotomy for ligation of persistent ductus
- Auscultation – inspiratory crackles and expiratory wheeze may be heard. If there is a loud second heart sound, pulmonary hypertension may have developed.

Extrapulmonary pathology
This is common and should be looked for specifically.

- Ventriculoperitoneal shunt – for acquired hydrocephalus secondary to intraventricular haemorrhage in the newborn period
- Inguinal herniae or scars following repair
- Blindness – retinopathy of prematurity or cortical blindness associated with periventricular leucomalacia
- Deafness
- Gastro-oesophageal reflux is common – look for vomit-streaked shoulders of parents!

Developmental assessment
- Milestones must be viewed in light of the corrected gestational age
- Delayed motor development may be exacerbated by:
  — failure to thrive with poor muscle bulk
  — chronic oxygen dependency
  — clinical rickets, which is be rare, although biochemical metabolic bone disease is common.

Neurological assessment
Ten per cent of infants born at less than 1500 g birthweight will have a major disability, e.g. blindness, deafness, cerebral palsy, global severe developmental delay.

MANAGEMENT

You would be expected to know the broad principles of management of this increasingly common condition.

Ventilation

Postnatal dexamethasone Postnatal dexamethasone is known to reduce the duration of ventilator dependency and recent meta-analysis indicates that early treatment with steroids significantly reduces the morbidity and mortality associated with chronic lung disease. However, steroid treatment is associated with a number of side-effects which must be considered, including increased risk of infection, hypertension, hyperglycaemia, spontaneous gastrointestinal haemorrhage or perforation and impaired antibody response to *Haemophilus influenzae* B immunization. Recent meta-analysis suggests that some systemic steroid regimens are associated with significantly increased neurodevelopmental risk of cerebral palsy.

Inhaled corticosteroids Inhaled steroids are usually tried as a 'systemic steroid-sparing treatment' when an infant with chronic lung disease cannot be weaned off dexamethasone without rebound increased oxygen requirement.

Diuretics The use of diuretics may result in short-term improvements in lung function but it is difficult to be sure that there are any long-term gains. Chronic furosemide (frusemide) administration is associated with hypercalcaemia which may lead to renal calcification.

Bronchodilators If, following discharge from hospital, the infant is repeatedly symptomatic with wheeze or is having repeated hospital admissions, a trial of nebulized bronchodilator (ipratropium bromide or salbutamol) is justified.

Nutrition

Perhaps the most important, but neglected, aspect of long-term treatment is to optimize nutrition, thereby improving somatic growth and lung growth. It may be necessary for feeds partly or wholly to be given by nasogastric tube at home, and carbohydrate, fat, folic acid, vitamin D and iron supplements may be indicated.

Emotional support

This is very important for the parents. Infants who have survived a long period of intensive care will generate anxieties in parents and GPs when they develop even trivial symptoms. There should be easy and ready access to a known paediatrician and the help of counsellors, therapists, specialist health visitors or family support nurses.

Intercurrent infections

These infants have a limited respiratory reserve and are more susceptible to infections, particularly respiratory syncytial virus (RSV) in the winter months. They require extra vigilance from parents and health care professionals, with a low threshold for admission.

SHORT CASES

CYANOSIS

- Anatomical right-to-left shunt
- Ventilation/perfusion mismatch
  — acute
  — severe asthma
  — bronchiolitis
  — pneumonia
  — chronic
  — CF
  — bronchiectasis
  — chronic lung fibrosis – fibrosing alveolitis
- Hypoventilation
  — central nervous system, e.g. acute coma
  — intercostal muscle weakness, e.g. congenital myopathy/muscular dystrophy
  — diaphragmatic weakness, e.g. acid maltase deficiency or phrenic nerve palsy
  — thoracic cage constriction, e.g. severe scoliosis
  — spinal cord injury
- Decreased inspired oxygen and rebreathing
- Methaemoglobinaemia.

OTHER SHORT CASES

Other short cases commonly encountered in the exam are listed below and will be dealt with in more detail in *Paediatric Short Cases for Postgraduate Examinations* by A Thomson, H Wallace and T Stephenson (Churchill Livingstone, Edinburgh, 2003):

- cystic fibrosis
- bronchiectasis, e.g. Kartagener's syndrome
- pneumonia
- pleural effusion
- chronic asthma
- chronic stridor
- fibrosing alveolitis.

INSPECTION

General well-being, nutritional status, dysmorphic features

In an infant, *do not undress* the patient until you know:

- respiratory rate
- colour
- nasal flaring, recession, accessory muscles
- stridor, wheeze

Hands – clubbing

Face – cyanosis, traumatic petechiae (coughing)

Neck – tracheal tug

Chest – deformity, scoliosis, Harrison's sulci, hyperinflation

Extras – oxygen, saturation monitors, inhalers, sputum pots, peak flow meters

PALPATION

Lymphadenopathy (neck and axilla) – can be done at the end

Feel for apex and trachea

Expansion

PERCUSSION (not in infant)

Compare both sides

Liver – upper border of the sixth intercostal space

AUSCULTATION

'I'm going to listen to your tummy.' Listen to child on mother's knee if possible

Breath sounds – vesicular, bronchial

Added sounds – crackles, wheeze

Vocal resonance

ANYTHING ELSE?

Liver – upper and lower borders

Measure PEFR: average PEFR (L/min) = (5 × height in cm) – 400

Third centile = average PEFR – 50

Check sputum pot

Plot height and weight on a growth chart appropriate for age and sex

ENT

The abdomen

5

Abdominal examination requires the child to be supine and adequately exposed. However, young children may find this frightening and be uncooperative, so you must try to make friends with the child whilst making your inspection and positioning him or her appropriately. Young children may be better examined on their mother's knee. Expose from the nipples to the knees unless the patient is a pubertal girl, and do not expose genitalia of older children.

INSPECTION

GENERAL

- Well or unwell – including conscious level (hepatic coma)
- Increased facial/body hair (ciclosporin side-effect)
- Skin rashes
  — dermatitis herpetiformis
  — perioral freckling (Peutz–Jeghers)
  — telangiectasia (Osler–Weber–Rendu)
- Pigmentation – remember, café-au-lait patches as a result of NF1 can present with gastrointestinal (GI) stromal tumours, with bleeding as a consequence and palpable abdominal masses, although these are very rare
- Dysmorphic features (mucopolysaccharidoses)
- Nutritional status – thriving or not thriving
- Nutritional support
  — nasogastric tube (long-term, short-term)
  — total parenteral nutrition (TPN): long-line, central line, portacath rarely used for home TPN
  — gastrostomy tube (PEG), button (French size and length are usually on the button itself)
  — peritoneal dialysis catheter
- Urinary catheter – spina bifida
- Older child in nappies – incontinent (neurological, behavioural problems)
- Race – more common, but not exclusively, in the following:
  — Afro-Caribbean: sickle cell disease
  — Asian or Cypriot (Mediterranean): thalassaemia
  — Chinese: hepatitis B.

HANDS

Finger clubbing
- Cystic fibrosis
- Crohn's disease and ulcerative colitis (extremely rare, not heard of in coeliac disease)
- Liver disease.

Anaemia
Look at nailbeds and palmar creases suggesting malabsorption or chronic gastrointestinal blood loss (recent acute haemorrhage is unlikely in the exam).

Koilonychia
● Iron deficiency – also look for smooth tongue and angular stomatitis
● Very rare in the UK.

Leuconychia
● Cirrhosis.

Xanthoma
● Hypercholesterolaemia (familial in children)
— tendon deposits
— tuberous xanthomas at elbows (calcification of older lesions can occur).

Palmar erythema
● Chronic liver disease
● Tremor (flapping classically).

FACE

Jaundice
● Look at sclera
● Is the patient's skin yellow or green/brown – characteristic of obstructive (cholestatic) jaundice?

Cyanosis/facial plethora
Plethora is often seen in chronic liver disease and cyanosis is seen in hepatopulmonary syndrome, where it results from extrapulmonary shunting. The patient may need oxygen and this is an indication for transplantation.

Spider naevi
● A cutaneous vascular malformation with a central arteriole supplying a number of radiating capillaries (Fig. 5.1)
● Pressure on the central arteriole blanches the whole spider. They are distributed over the area that is drained by the superior vena cava. More than three is a significant number in prepubertal children (occasionally, more may be seen in girls without any underlying abnormality)
● Chronic liver disease (excess oestrogens)
● Telangiectasia, as in:
— Osler–Weber–Rendu syndrome
— ataxic telangiectasia.

MOUTH

● Pigmentation – Peutz–Jeghers syndrome (perioral and buccal pigmentation)
● Ulcers
— aphthous ulcers
— Crohn's disease, ulcerative colitis, coeliac, Behçet's disease

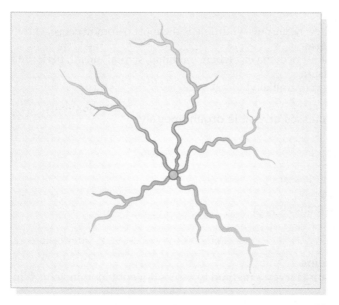

Fig. 5.1 Spider naevus.

- Dental caries – chronic vomiting, coeliac disease
- Gum hypertrophy (gingival changes)
  — myeloid leukaemia
  — drugs: ciclosporin, phenytoin
- Macroglossia – in Down's syndrome, the tongue rolls forward but there is not true macroglossia. There are five important causes of macroglossia:
  — hypothyroidism
  — Beckwith–Wiedemann syndrome (look for linear fissures on the ear lobe)
  — mucopolysaccharidoses
  — Pompé's glycogen storage disease
  — amyloid (usually adults).

ABDOMEN

Distension
Is the distension:

- central or flank
- symmetrical or asymmetrical
- generalized or localized?

Remember the *five Fs* (also organomegaly):

- Fat
- Faeces
  — Hirschsprung's disease
  — constipation
- Flatus
  — air swallowing
  — malabsorption, e.g. coeliac disease; intestinal obstruction is unlikely in an exam

- Fluid
  - ascites: nephrotic syndrome is the most common cause; chronic liver disease
  - look for oedema elsewhere: pretibial, scrotal, sacral, periorbital, pleural effusion
- Fetus – very unlikely!

Obvious masses or visible organomegaly

Scars
Don't forget:

- renal angle scars
- liver biopsy
- laparascopic surgery.

Striae

Dilated veins
Use William Harvey's method to assess flow of blood in veins (Fig. 5.2).

Caput medusae Veins drain *away from the umbilicus* due to portal vein obstruction. If present, then look for other signs of liver disease (liver failure is a specific end-stage problem), e.g. liver flap of the hands.

Superior vena cava (SVC) obstruction (Fig. 5.2) Blood flows *inferiorly* in the superficial abdominal veins (look for this in children with central lines, complication thereof, although rare).

Inferior vena cava (IVC) obstruction (Fig. 5.2) Blood flows *superiorly* in superficial abdominal veins (obstruction is unlikely in exams).

Stomas
- Ileostomy versus colostomy (position)
- Mucous fistula
- Caecostomy tube for antegrade enemas in some children with chronic constipation (the so-called MACE procedure, or Malone antegrade colonic enema).

Genitalia/perianal area
You must at least offer to examine if Crohn's, ulcerative colitis or Behçet's is suspected, looking for fissures or skin tags. You should inspect the genitalia of an infant without being specifically invited to do so by the examiner:

- ambiguous (see Ch. 6)
- undescended testis – if you suspect the child has an undescended testis, first examine the scrotum with the child standing, then lying and finally, if you are still uncertain, in a squatting position (which abolishes the cremasteric reflex in cases of retractile testes).

Herniae/scrotal swellings
- Umbilical hernia
  - common in healthy Afro-Caribbeans below 5 years of age
  - prematurity
  - Down's syndrome

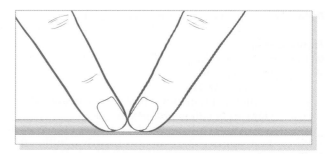

1. Press on veins with two fingers

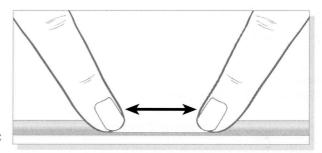

2. Pull fingers apart

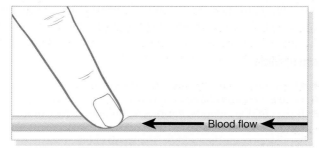

3. Lift one finger — does vein fill?

Blood flow

Fig. 5.2 William Harvey test: to determine flow of blood in veins.

— hypothyroidism
— mucopolysaccharidoses
● Inguinal hernia
● Hydrocele.

Skin

Scratch marks
● Obstructive (cholestatic) jaundice
● Lichenification
● Excoriation
● Erythema
● Visible pruritus may be evident on inspection of the patient.

Bruising
● Liver dysfunction
● Haematological disease.

Rash   Dermatitis herpetiformis in coeliac disease.

Pigmentation
- Depigmentation (vitiligo)
- Hyperpigmentation
  — café-au-lait patches
  — incontinentia pigmentosa (not so rare in exams!)
    — stage III of cutaneous lesions
    — associated with dystrophic changes of hair, nails, teeth
    — from approx 12–24 months to early adulthood
- Hypopigmentation
  — incontinentia pigmentation (stage IV of cutaneous lesions)
    — permanent linear hypopigmented streaks
    — particularly on legs
    — associated with alopecia.

Nappy
In infants, examine the urine and stool at this stage.

PALPATION

NECK

Don't forget to check for lymphadenopathy, especially if there is splenomegaly, but this can be left until the end.

ABDOMEN

- *Do not* take your eyes off the child's face.
- Ensure that your hands are warm.
- If the child is anxious, various techniques can be employed to help relax the abdominal muscles:
  — place on mother's knee, if a small child
  — reposition: get the child to flex his/her hips and place the feet on a couch
  — make a game of it: ask the child to blow out his/her tummy and try to touch your hand. Now ask him/her to suck the tummy in (this is looking for peritonism). Ask the child to help you by placing your hand over their hand and feeling the tummy together.

Gentle palpation
- Tell the child what you are going to do and ask if the tummy is sore anywhere.
- Begin with gentle palpation to detect any obvious abnormality and to help the child relax.
- Be gentle: feel with your hand flat on the abdomen and fingers flexed at the metacarpophalangeal joints.
- Be methodical: begin away from you and examine each quadrant in turn.

Deep palpation
- Now repeat the sequence and palpate more deeply.
- Tenderness is unlikely in the exam but, if found, you must detect:
  — location of tenderness
  — guarding: voluntary/involuntary
  — rebound tenderness.

Organ palpation (Table 5.1)

Liver Flex the fingers at the metacarpophalangeal joint, using the forefingers parallel to the costal margin. Begin in the right iliac fossa and work up towards the costal margin. Children frequently have a palpable liver edge (up to 2 cm). If hepatomegaly is present, describe:

● position – measure the liver edge below the costal margin in the midclavicular line with a tape measure, although time is often limited and examiners are unlikely to object if you report it in finger breadths and offer to measure
● texture
— smooth or nodular
— firm or soft
● whether tender – was it uncomfortable on palpation?
● whether pulsatile – hepatic AV malformation (very rare in the UK)
● whether expansile – tricuspid incompetence (very rare in the UK)
● percussion – don't forget to define the upper border of the liver to exclude hyperinflation as the cause of the palpable liver edge. Specify the upper border by counting the rib spaces.

Spleen
● Palpate from the right iliac fossa with the left hand splinting the lower edge of the rib cage posteriorly.
● If there is difficulty, lie the child on his/her right side and palpate with the child taking deep breaths.
● The spleen tip may be palpable in normal neonates.
● Measure the spleen from the costal margin in the midclavicular line.
● Percuss out the borders of the spleen.

Kidneys *Bimanual palpation* – push up with the left hand in the renal angle (the costovertebral angle) and feel the kidney anteriorly with the right hand. Ballot kidneys between hands. A common mistake made by candidates is to push too laterally with their left hand.

Masses If a mass is found, remember to describe:

● site, size, shape
● consistency – faeces are indentible
● mobility – does it move on respiration?
● whether tender

Table 5.1 Differentiation of organomegaly

	Liver	Spleen	Kidneys
Site of enlargement	To RIF	To RIF	Flanks
Inspiration	Descends	Descends	Descends
Can get above it?	No	No	Yes
Special features	None	Notch	Ballotable
Percussion	Dull	Dull	Resonant (overlying bowel)
Pulsatile	May be	No	No
Expansile	May be	No	No

RIF, right iliac fossa

● whether pulsatile – abdominal aneurysms are very rare in children
● percussion – is it dull or is there bowel overlying it?
● does it alter after micturition/defaecation?

PERCUSSION

Percuss for the following unless the child is uncooperative:

● organomegaly
● mass
● fluid.

ASCITES

Examine for ascites if:

● there is hepatomegaly (very likely also to have splenomegaly)
● there are any other signs of liver disease – clubbing, palmar erythema, spider naevi, jaundice, prominent periumbilical veins
● the abdomen appears distended
● there is oedema apparent elsewhere.

To demonstrate ascites, test for shifting dullness and a fluid thrill, involving the examiner in the latter. The test for shifting dullness is shown in Figure 5.3. In the supine position, free fluid, which is dull to percussion, gravitates to the lowest part of the abdomen, and the gut, which contains resonant gas, floats upwards. Percussion from the umbilicus towards the flanks reveals a line of demarcation where the resonance of the bowel gas becomes the dullness of the free fluid. The position at which this occurs should be marked. If the patient is then rolled over onto the side, the fluid moves to the lower flank and the line of demarcation between dullness and resonance shifts (see below). In gross ascites, the abdomen is generally distended, the umbilicus is everted, the flanks are especially full, and the scrotum is full. The skin may also be oedematous.

AUSCULTATION

BOWEL SOUNDS

Listen for bowel sounds if the abdomen is distended or the child has a nasogastric tube.

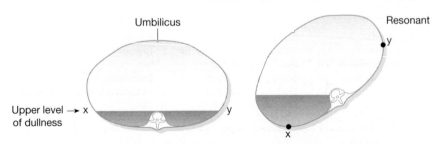

Fig. 5.3 To test for ascites using the shifting dullness technique.

RENAL BRUITS

Listening for renal bruits is not a routine part of the examination, but should be done if the child is hypertensive or has neurofibromatosis, as these are associated with renal artery stenosis.

GENITALIA

TESTES

For a male infant:

- check to see if the testes are descended
- ensure that the urethral meatus is in the normal position.

SCROTAL SWELLING (inguinal hernia/hydrocele – Table 5.2)

- It is important to establish the landmarks, although most inguinal herniae in children are indirect.
- Examine the patient lying down initially, and then re-examine standing up if old enough and if you are uncertain.

ANYTHING ELSE?

ANUS/RECTUM

Offer to examine the anus and rectum if this is relevant, e.g. in a child with inflammatory bowel disease for fissures, skin tags, fistulae and excoriation.

GROWTH

Plot height and weight on a centile chart appropriate for age and sex. Think about nutrition issues and mention skin folds for body fat stores (triceps usually measured) and mid-arm circumference (for muscle bulk).

URINE/STOOL

Look at an infant's nappy if you have not already done so, especially if jaundiced, and offer to check the urine of an older child if relevant.

Table 5.2 Hernia versus hydrocele

Differentiating features	Hernia	Hydrocele
Transmits cough impulse?	Yes	No
Can get you above it?	No	Yes
Can testis be palpated separately?	Yes	No
Transillumination	No	Yes

COMMON LONG CASES

- Coeliac disease
- Inflammatory bowel disease
- Biliary atresia (post-Kasai, usually, or post-liver transplant)
- Chronic renal failure

COELIAC DISEASE

Coeliac disease is a gluten-sensitive enteropathy characterized by varying degrees of villous atrophy in genetically susceptible individuals, over 90% of whom are positive for the HLA DQ2 haplotype. It is due to an intolerance of the gliadin fraction of dietary gluten. In the majority of patients, it is responsive to a lifelong gluten-free diet. It has an incidence of 1 in 200, when population screening is adopted. There is much geographical variability. Prior to screening of populations, the prevalence was 1 in 2000 (when one investigates symptomatic patients).

HISTORY

Onset of symptoms
- Were the symptoms related to age of weaning onto solids (usually 4–6 months in the UK)?
- Classical presentation is within the first 2 years of life. In the UK, as with other countries (e.g. Finland), presentation is tending to be later in childhood.

Symptoms

In a young child with a classical presentation
- Diarrhoea – classically offensive, pale, frequent, bulky stools of malabsorption
- Failure to thrive
- Vomiting and weight loss
- Anorexia
- Short stature
- Abdominal distension
- Constipation is present in up to 10% in some series.

In an older child
- Less specific features – recurrent abdominal pains, lethargy, nausea, etc., but may well have same symptoms
- Anaemia (predominantly iron deficiency +/– folate)
- Growth failure
- Pubertal delay.

Developmental milestones
They may have delayed motor milestones.

Dietary changes
- Parents are often struck by the improvement in the child's temperament on a gluten-free diet. Many people who consider themselves asymptomatic realize they have been unwell when they go gluten-free.

- Are the parents aware of which foods to avoid?
- Have they seen a dietician?
- Do they get regular dietary follow-up?
- Do they know which cereals contain gluten and also that many commercially available rusks and baby foods are gluten-free?
- Recent evidence is in support of allowing oats (oat 'gliadin' is relatively non-toxic compared with wheat, barley, rye, etc.).

Support
Are the parents in touch with any support groups such as the Coeliac Society (membership is free to registered coeliacs)?

EXAMINATION

The examination may be normal if the patient is already on a gluten-free diet.

Classical presentation
- Anaemia
- Lassitude, apathy, miserable
- Distended abdomen
- Wasted buttocks.

Acute classical presentation of coeliac disease is rare but examiners will expect you to comment on what the expected clinical features of presentation would have been.

Other features include:
- Short stature
- Glossitis, angular stomatitis
- Dermatitis herpetiformis – erythematous papules with excoriation +/– vesicles (very rarely seen, but seen on extensor surfaces: knees, buttocks, elbows)
- Delayed puberty
- Rickets – swollen wrists and costochondral joints due to malabsorption of fat-soluble vitamin D
- Aphthous ulcers.

NB. Remember, many coeliacs are found through screening in at-risk groups and may be mono- or asymptomatic, but are nonetheless coeliac.

INVESTIGATIONS

Some of the investigations you should be able to discuss are outlined below.

Autoantibodies
Remember, selective IgA deficiency is associated with coeliac disease and may be the cause of a false-negative coeliac screen (as the standard antibodies are IgA versions).

Antigliadin antibodies (AGAs) There are IgA and IgG versions of AGA. They are detected by the ELISA test, given in units/mL. There is variable sensitivity and specificity from laboratory to laboratory. The IgA AGA test has good specificity and sensitivity, whereas the IgG AGA has good sensitivity but poor specificity (false-positive IgG in cow's milk protein intolerance, Crohn's and postinfective states; false-positive IgA in atopic eczema, pemphigus, pemphigoid). Remember, IgA deficiency occurs in 1 in 50 of patients with coeliac disease, hence the need to check IgA level and request IgG versions of the tests.

Antiendomysial antibodies (EmAs)   This is the current gold standard test. It is a qualitative test which shows immunofluorescence within connective tissue of smooth muscle and is consequently dependent on the experience of the observer. It is now performed on human umbilical cord. IgA and IgG versions are both performed. Sensitivity and specificity are over 95% in adults. The test is less sensitive in children under 2 years, where the false-negative rate is higher, depending on the experience of the observer.

Anti-tissue transglutaminase antibodies (tTGs)   Tissue transglutaminase is an enzyme involved in mucosal inflammation and healing, and is the antigen to which EmAs are directed. First described in 1997, this is a quantitative ELISA test, for both IgA and IgG versions, which is better suited for mass screening. It has good specificity and sensitivity, approaching that of EmA, and is becoming more widely available.

Antibodies are a good way of screening but will not replace intestinal biopsy which remains essential for diagnosis. Antibodies such as EmA will usually normalize at around a year after a strict gluten-free diet.

Intestinal biopsy

Most centres now perform a small-bowel biopsy endoscopically. The technique of capsule biopsy should still be known, however. A normal jejunal biopsy in a patient receiving a normal gluten intake excludes coeliac disease at that point in time. It may be, however, that the patient may develop it in future (so-called latent coeliacs). In the infant with chronic diarrhoea, assay of disaccharidase levels can exclude disaccharidase deficiency, giardiasis or bacterial overgrowth. This can be investigated by examination of the duodenal juice, and a number of rare conditions, which have characteristic appearances (e.g. intestinal lymphangiectasia, abetalipoproteinaemia and other rarer enteropathies such as autoimmune enteropathy, tufting enteropathy and microvillus inclusion disease), can also be looked for. Contraindications to endoscopic biopsy include a bleeding diathesis (vitamin K malabsorption), intercurrent illness and a severely debilitated infant in whom perforation of the small bowel may occur. You should be able to describe how you would perform a biopsy and interpret the results.

MANAGEMENT

- Gluten-free diet for life
- Dietician involvement is essential to educate the parents on foods to be avoided and purchasing of gluten-free products and to ensure good calcium intake
- Follow-up – lifelong review of these patients is required with prompt investigation of new symptoms and blood test abnormalities.

DISCUSSION

Criteria for diagnosis/need for re-challenge biopsy (ESPGAN criteria 1990)

Current European guidelines stipulate that children under 2 years shown to have villous atrophy on biopsy, should be re-challenged and biopsied some time after the initial diagnosis. One biopsy in those over 2 years is considered sufficient if there is a compatible history, serological evidence, compatible histology and obvious clinical and serological response to a gluten-free diet.

Pathophysiology The immunological mechanisms underlying this disorder are complex but involve T-cell presentation of fragments of alpha-gliadin, which mediates the inflammatory response in the lamina propria and epithelium. Genetic predisposition to developing gluten intolerance is well established and certain haplotypes have been associated with increased susceptibility: B8, DR3 and DQ2, DR5/DR7 and DQ2 and DR4 and DQ8 alleles. Other non-HLA genes may be involved. Siblings and offspring of patients with coeliac disease have a 10% risk of developing the disease themselves. Screening at-risk groups may be appropriate: family members, type 1 diabetics, autoimmune hepatitis, thyroiditis, Addison's, Sjögren's, Down's syndrome, Turner's syndrome, Williams syndrome, those with selective IgA deficiency.

Differential diagnosis of an abnormal jejunal biopsy

Dietary
- Coeliac disease
- Transient gluten intolerance
- Cow's milk sensitive enteropathy
- Soy protein intolerance
- Protein energy malnutrition.

Infection
- Gastroenteritis and postgastroenteritis syndromes
- Giardiasis
- Tropical sprue.

Immune disorders
- Autoimmune enteropathy
- Acquired hypogammaglobulinaemia
- Severe combined immunodeficiency.

Drugs
- Chemotherapy.

Long-term complications and their relationship to compliance with a gluten-free diet

- Ulcerative jejunoileitis
- Enteropathy-associated T-cell lymphoma (EATCL)
- Carcinoma of pharynx, oesophagus, colon and rectum
- Organ-specific autoimmunity (thyroid, adrenal, pancreas).

Other topics

- The effect of the disease on the child and the family
- How and when do you approach the discussion of the long-term complications of the disease with the patient?
- What is the value of continued outpatient surveillance?

CHRONIC INFLAMMATORY BOWEL DISEASE (IBD)

Crohn's and ulcerative colitis (UC) are not uncommon long cases in the clinical exam. There are a number of important physical signs to be elicited by the candidate but success will depend largely on your ability to take a good history, gain a reasonable rapport with the patient and discuss sensibly the practical management of the disease as well as the patient and family.

HISTORY

Mode of presentation
Around 20% of IBD presents in childhood (under 18 years). Crohn's and UC represent a spectrum of chronic IBD conditions that present in protean ways and are accompanied by a variety of systemic sequelae. Crohn's disease is a transmural, segmental chronic inflammatory disease affecting any part of the gut from the mouth to the anus, in contrast to ulcerative colitis which is a recurrent continuous inflammatory disease involving the mucosal and submucosal layers of the rectum with variable proximal extension up the large bowel. Consequently, a history of lower bowel symptoms without symptoms suggestive of involvement higher up the intestine is more suggestive of UC. Constitutional symptoms are much more likely in Crohn's.

Crohn's disease is on the increase, with an incidence of 3 per 100 000, and UC is very constant with an incidence of 0.7 per 100 000. It is more common in families, with a lifetime risk of around 10%. It is also more common in Jewish populations, from middle European extraction. Maternal and passive smoking increase the risk of Crohn's. Inheritance is polygenic, with putative susceptibility genes from linkage studies showing higher numbers of patients with markers on chromosomes 1, 3, 6, 7, 10, 12, 22 and X (increased risk in Turner's syndrome). There is also a high twin concordance.

Presentation can be remarkably variable but a rough guide is as follows:

- *Crohn's* – anorexia, weight loss, abdominal pain, diarrhoea (bloody, with mucus), growth failure, pubertal delay
- *Ulcerative colitis* – weight loss, abdominal pain, rectal bleeding, diarrhoea/urgency.

Current symptoms

Investigations
What investigations has the child undergone so far and why?

Operations
Has the child required any surgery for the IBD?

Drug history
- Medication tried previously – reasons for discontinuing drugs
- Current medication
- In an older child, who gives local, rectal treatment?
- Complications of medication.

Extraintestinal manifestations of the disease
These are similar for both groups:

- uveitis
- arthralgia
- skin manifestations
  — erythema nodosum
  — pyoderma gangrenosum
- liver disease (sclerosing cholangitis, autoimmune hepatitis, gallstones in Crohn's)
- renal disease (stones)
- growth retardation/delayed puberty/retarded bone age.

Dietary history
- Studies have shown that patients with IBD may only ingest 50–80% of their recommended daily calorie requirement, usually because of pain precipitated by eating; therefore nutritional supplements may be required to optimize growth.
- Are episodes exacerbated by certain foods (milk, wheat, others)?
- Has the child required a period of total parenteral nutrition or nasogastric (or G-tube) feeding?

Impact on patient/family
How has this chronic disease, characterized as it is by exacerbations and relapses, affected the child and the family?

- How much school has been missed?
- How does the child manage at school (toileting, episodes of diarrhoea, pain)?
- What compromises, if any, has the family made for the child's benefit?
- What effect has this illness had on the other children in the family?
- Are there, perhaps, emotional and psychological problems with brothers and sisters who may resent the extra attention being lavished by friends, relations and professionals on the patient?
- How much insight into the condition does the child have? Clearly this will depend on the age of the child, and while it would be unwise to mention directly some of the more worrisome complications, e.g. malignancy (ulcerative colitis), the examiners may expect you to have gleaned something about the child's own understanding of what the future holds.

EXAMINATION

Presentation is dependent on disease distribution and severity.

Is the child well or unwell?

Nutritional status/growth
Growth data are essential; you will be provided with the necessary charts. Assessment of nutritional status is clearly important and should prompt you to measure skinfold thicknesses (if skinfold calipers are available), triceps skin fold, mid-arm circumference (and head circumference, not usually for nutritional status, but for general growth).

PASS

The abdomen

Abdominal examination

Carry out with particular reference to:

- localized or generalized tenderness
- masses
- scars
- stomas
- gastrostomy tube
- perioral – mouth ulcers
- anal and perianal region – pendulous skin tags, fistulae, fissures, abscesses
- anaemia
- hypoalbuminaemia
- evidence of liver dysfunction.

Extraintestinal manifestations

- Skin – erythema nodosum, pyoderma gangrenosum
- Eyes – conjunctivitis, episcleritis, uveitis
- Arthritis – monoarticular, ankylosing spondylitis, sacroileitis
- Hepatobiliary – cirrhosis, gallstones, sclerosing cholangitis, pericholangitis, renal disease (stones).

Complications of medication

- Steroids
- Metronidazole (peripheral neuropathy)
- ASA (acetyl salicylic acid) – headaches, rashes, diarrhoea!

INVESTIGATIONS

Radiological

Left wrist X-ray Bone age can be delayed (usually in Crohn's disease).

Plain abdominal X-ray In the acute situation (when toxic megacolon is suspected) this may reveal evidence of obstruction or dilatation, thickening of bowel wall or stones.

Abdominal ultrasound scan This is good at detecting small- and large-bowel wall thickening, nodal enlargement, abscesses, stones and fistulae.

Barium meal and follow-through (some use small-bowel enema [enteroclysis] via nasoduodenal tube) Vital in order to assess small-bowel involvement in Crohn's. Typically in Crohn's disease the mucosa is described as showing a patchily involved small bowel with cobblestone-like pattern, the bowel wall is thickened, the loops separated and there may be evidence of fistula formation. The presence of skip lesions, lumen narrowing, thickening and fissuring ('rose-thorn ulcers') is typical of Crohn's (may be seen in chronic granulomatous disease so be wary of saying they are characteristic).

A barium meal may be performed to detect the presence of gastric and oesophageal varices which may develop as a complication of hepatic involvement and portal hypertension. As well as being seen on ultrasound scan, these are readily diagnosed and treated by upper endoscopy and banding/injection sclerotherapy.

Barium enema This is seldom performed, as endoscopy would precede this for diagnosis and is the investigation of choice in acute colitis. In ulcerative colitis a barium enema usually shows a diffuse continuous distal lesion confined to the rectum and colon. Not the investigation of choice.

White cell scan This is not a first-line investigation. Indium-labelled leucocyte scans have been used to assess the extent of active disease but the technique involves a relatively high radiation exposure and should only be used in carefully selected circumstances (such as the differentiation of an acute vs. chronic stricture in terminal ileal Crohn's disease).

Endoscopy procedures Paediatric colonoscopy is now performed in most teaching hospital settings by specially trained gastroenterologists. This allows a view of the mucosal appearance of the whole of the colon, including the terminal ileum, and biopsy of the mucosa is performed routinely from all areas whether 'normal appearing' or not. Bowel preparation is mandatory, usually given by mouth rather than enema, using medications such as sodium picosulphate, oral phosphate solution and lavage via nasogastric tube with Kleen Prep. Polyps can be snared and strictures dilated if found at endoscopy. As part of the diagnostic work-up, upper endoscopy may help to differentiate Crohn's from UC with the presence of characteristic histological changes on biopsy of the upper GI tract.

Haematology/clinical chemistry
- Anaemia – iron deficiency anaemia is common
- White cell count may be raised and neutrophils elevated
- Acute-phase reactants – erythrocyte sedimentation rate (ESR) and C-reactive protein (CRP) can be measured as a way of monitoring disease activity
- Thrombocytosis and hypoalbuminaemia are also commonly found and can be used to monitor progress
- Liver function tests may be deranged
- In acute colitis, prolonged diarrhoea may cause dehydration, hypokalaemia and acidosis.

Genetic susceptibility studies
See p. 89.

DISCUSSION

The approach to management
IBD is a chronic paediatric disease that requires treatment by a multidisciplinary team of experts (doctor, nurse, dietician, social worker, psychologist, pharmacist, biochemist, microbiologist) which depends on patient cooperation from the outset.

The aims of management are:

- to induce and maintain remission
- to maintain adequate nutrition
- to treat complications
- to optimize quality of life
- to educate the patient, family and school and provide support.

Medical management

Induction of remission

Nutritional therapy   Aggressive enteral nutritional therapy (previously elemental feeds, but now there is a move back to whole protein feeds) is effective in inducing remission in Crohn's disease (usually small-bowel disease patients) in up to 70–80% of cases.

Steroids
- Induce remission in >80% of Crohn's disease
- Oral prednisolone 1 mg/kg/day, up to a maximum 60 mg/day (most children maximum 40 mg), gradually tapered after remission is gained, usually after 4 weeks; tapered by 5 mg each week
- Topical steroids – liquid, or more usually foam, enemas for disease confined to left side of colon, rectum and sigmoid colon (splenic flexure accessed by good technique)
- Budesonide can be used as an enema in active distal ulcerative colitis or as a delayed-release tablet in Crohn's and reduces systemic side-effects, but there is some question as to efficacy and we don't have good experience with it.

Systemic steroids
- In severe cases, intravenous treatment is required
- Intravenous hydrocortisone 1 mg/kg four times daily (some use 24-hour infusion)
- Newer corticosteroids, such as budesonide, may be less toxic than the older agents such as prednisolone.

Antibiotics
- Broad-spectrum antibiotics (cefotaxime and metronidazole, or ampicillin, gentamicin and metronidazole) may be used when a colitic presents acutely, as there may be abscess or bacterial translocation in the inflamed gut, but the majority use no antibiotics unless there are specific worries (many IBD patients are febrile but are culture-negative).
- Metronidazole is effective in terminal ileal and particularly perianal disease, although peripheral neuropathy may develop with long-term use. Often, ciprofloxacin is used in addition to metronidazole, usually in a 2–3 month course.

Immunomodulators   These drugs are used for patients who either do not respond to steroids or who respond but seem to be dependent on steroids (those who flare on tapering), and have been shown to have benefit in both Crohn's and UC.
- Azathioprine (usually the next choice after steroids; dose up to 2 mg/kg/day) – some use 6-mercaptopurine, of which azathioprine is prodrug. Generally used for a minimum of 4 years when started
- Ciclosporin/tacrolimus – may be used as a 'rescue' drug intravenously in acute colitis (UC and Crohn's), with 50% gaining remission, but many tend to relapse after discontinuation. It has been associated with increased BP, hypomagnesaemia, seizures. Needs drug level monitoring, PCP prophylaxis
- 6-mercaptopurine (mentioned above)
- Methotrexate (used after azathioprine if no response, either orally or usually subcutaneously once weekly).

New drugs   Infliximab (anti-TNF-alpha) – tumour necrosis factor (TNF) is a major proinflammatory cytokine. This antibody (human/mouse chimera) is useful in Crohn's disease (possibly UC, trials started) and has been shown to heal disease and close fistulas. Given as an infusion, the usual treatment course is three to four, but others give multiple infusions to maintain remission.

Maintaining remission

Steroids
- There is no evidence to suggest that low-dose steroid therapy can maintain remission in Crohn's disease.
- Associated with significant toxicity in chronic use.

5-Aminosalicylates Some start ASA at same time as steroids, while others wait until 4 weeks when hopefully remission is gained. Particularly effective in UC.
- Sulfasalazine – 5-aminosalicylate and sulfapyridine, first available preparation for 70 years
- Mesalazine – 5-aminosalicylate, e.g. Asacol, Salofalk, both pH-dependent, delayed-release preparations, start dispersing in distal ileum; Pentasa starts in upper GI tract
- ASA preparations have shown marginal long-term benefit for remission maintenance in Crohn's and are used in both Crohn's and UC.

Surgical management

Acute emergency
- Severe fulminating disease not responding to medical therapy
- Toxic megacolon.

Non-acute situation
- Growth failure and/or debilitating symptoms despite intensive and prolonged medical therapy in the face of stricture terminal ileum and episodes of obstruction or subacute obstruction.
- Colectomy – curative in UC. A pouch operation is usually performed as part of the initial procedure or as a two-stage procedure. Most Crohn's patients will require at least one operation at some point, although surgery is less effective in Crohn's due to recurrence elsewhere in the gut.
- Prevention of malignancy in long-standing UC. Risk factors – disease extent, severity and duration (remember, CD also has malignant potential). Surveillance colonoscopy usually carried out from 8 to 10 years after diagnosis.

Long-term prognosis
Most IBD patients suffer relapsing episodes of varying severity: some have mild disease and are seldom troubled, whereas some have very debilitating disease requiring multiple surgery, sometimes ending with short gut syndrome and lifelong parenteral nutrition dependence. Crohn's is associated with an increased risk of cancer, but regular colonoscopic surveillance as in UC is not yet advocated.

Current theories regarding the pathogenesis of chronic IBD
- The role of infection and/or a cell-mediated hypersensitivity reaction
- Abnormality of T cells

- Genetic problem of immune tolerance – balancing act of pro- and anti-inflammatory cytokines: T-cell response/macrophages → increased cytokines/TNF-1 → granuloma.

Effect on growth

- In one recent study, growth was impaired in >50% of cases, with approximately 25% of cases falling in the category of short stature. However, endocrine function tests demonstrate normal growth hormone secretion.
- Typical pattern is of growth retardation associated with delayed skeletal maturation.
- Cytokines have a deleterious effect on the cartilage growth plate and patients have been shown to have reduced levels of IGF-1.
- Puberty is also delayed in a significant number.

BILIARY ATRESIA (EXTRAHEPATIC BILIARY ATRESIA, EHBA)

Biliary atresia has an incidence of 1 in 15 000 live births with a slight female predominance. It is an idiopathic disorder resulting in obliteration of the biliary tract (Landing's theory of ductal plate abnormalities) with consequent chronic liver failure and death unless surgical intervention is performed. It is the leading indication for liver transplantation in children. Biliary atresia accounts for approximately one-third of infant cholestasis and must be ruled out in any infant presenting with conjugated jaundice. There are two forms:

Fetal

- 10–35% of cases
- No jaundice-free interval after physiological jaundice
- Associated with congenital problems (?prenatal insult) – polysplenia, asplenia, cardiac abnormalities, renal, other GI problems.

Perinatal

- 65–90%
- Presents at 4–8 weeks of age with cholestasis and jaundice (ask and look for stool colour)
- Usually full term
- May be a jaundice-free interval
- Pathogenesis (several theories postulated but no solid evidence):
  — genetic (but many discordant identical twins)
  — infection (reovirus type 3, CMV, EBV, rotavirus)
  — ischaemic injury
  — immunological
    — HLA class I abnormalities
    — ANCA positivity (ANCA-positive in adults with sclerosing cholangitis and autoimmune hepatitis)
    — abnormal embryological biliary development suggested by mouse model with possible bile duct cells remodelling, the ductal plate theory
  — vascular injury.

EXAMINATION

A jaundiced infant may have no liver enlargement and look extremely well! Look for dysmorphisms (Alagille, etc.).

INVESTIGATIONS

Stools/urine
- Test for bilirubin
- Exclude congenital infection
- Exclude urinary tract infection.

Biochemistry/serology
- Abnormal liver function tests – predominantly alkaline phosphatase (ALP) and γ-glutamyl transpeptidase (GGT), but also alanine/aspartate aminotransferase (ALT/AST).
- Conjugated jaundice and elevated total bilirubin
- Check albumin and coagulation
- Exclude genetic causes – α-1-antitrypsin deficiency, cystic fibrosis
- Exclude metabolic disorder – urine and plasma amino acids
- Exclude infection – congenital and hepatitis.

Ultrasound scan of bile ducts and gall bladder
- May be contracted, normal or not seen
- Bile ducts may be dilated (choledochal cyst).

Isotope scan
Perform an isotope scan, to look at liver uptake and excretion.

Percutaneous liver biopsy
Usually performed after 4 weeks, by which time bile duct proliferation will be apparent, if present. Before 4 weeks of age, biopsy may show non-specific changes and be falsely misleading. Liver biopsy demonstrates features of extrahepatic biliary obstruction: proliferation, cholestasis, periportal oedema and fibrosis.

TREATMENT

Treatment consists of surgical bypass of the fibrotic ducts: Kasai portoenterostomy, with Roux loop of small bowel anastomosed to the ductal remnant and the atretic segment excised. If surgery is performed before 60 days, 80% of children will achieve bile drainage. This does not, however, guarantee success, as irreversible fibrosis may have developed following the onset of cholestasis and the child may go on to require transplant anyway. The success rate decreases with advancing age. Surgery is best performed in a centre with an experienced surgeon who regularly carries out such procedures.

PROGNOSIS

Rule of thirds:

- One-third fail and need transplant within a year
- One-third require a liver by teenage years
- One-third avoid transplant (but may have chronic liver disease).

Associated problems
- Cholestasis
  - nutritional
  - vitamin deficiency (including bleeding issues – vitamin K)
  - malabsorption (need for MCT-based feeding)
- Poor growth
- Pruritus/excoriation
- Xanthomas
- Portal hypertension/varices/bleeding
- Avoiding aspirin and NSAIDs.

Longer-term problems
- Hepatorenal syndrome
- Hepatopulmonary syndrome and ascites
- Hypoalbuminaemia
- Infection
- Liver failure and ultimately transplant.

CHRONIC RENAL FAILURE

Chronic renal failure is rare in childhood but is not uncommonly encountered in the clinical exam. In childhood, chronic renal failure is secondary to a number of causes, and congenital and familial causes are more common than acquired diseases. Most children will have had their renal disease detected before birth by antenatal ultrasound scan or will have previously identified renal disease.

HISTORY

How did the problem present?

Antenatal diagnosis? Ultrasound scan before birth can detect renal abnormalities, which may have come to light due to oligohydramnios:

- congenital dysplasia
- renal obstruction – posterior urethral valves in boys.

Underlying disease
- Structural malformation of the kidney (may/may not be detected antenatally)
  - renal hypoplasia/dysplasia
  - reflux nephropathy
- Glomerular diseases
  - Henoch–Schönlein purpura
  - idiopathic glomerulonephritis
- Vascular diseases – haemolytic uraemic syndrome
- . Genetically inherited diseases – cystinosis
- Systemic diseases – SLE.

Symptomatic renal failure
Symptoms rarely develop before renal function deteriorates to less than 50% of normal, but may present with:

- lethargy and anorexia
- failure to thrive/poor growth

- delayed puberty
- polydypsia/polyuria
- bony deformities of renal osteodystrophy
- hypertension.

Incidental finding
Rarely, chronic renal failure can be picked up on routine blood test or proteinuria.

EXAMINATION

- Growth – plot height and weight (which will be provided) on an appropriate chart
- Nutritional status – appetite is usually poor and patients require supplementation
- Blood pressure
- Anaemia
- Scars
  — biopsy
  — transplant – iliac fossa scar (Rutherford Morrison scar)
- Fistulae – some patients may be on haemodialysis and have an AV fistula in their forearm
- Peritoneal dialysis catheters – ask about dialysis and previous catheter infections
- Bony abnormalities
  — rickets
  — splayed metaphysis
- Nutritional support
  — nasogastric tube
  — gastrostomy tube.

MANAGEMENT

This requires coordination of the various members of the multidisciplinary team to ensure that the following aims are achieved:

- prevention of symptoms and metabolic/endocrine abnormalities associated with renal failure
- optimization of growth and development
- preservation of residual renal function.

Nutrition
Adequate calorie intake is essential.

- Anorexia and vomiting are common.
- In young children under 2 years, normal calorie and protein requirements are two to three times greater/kg than in adults and this must be adjusted to ensure adequate growth, but watch for accumulation of toxic metabolites.
- Supplementation is usually required – vitamin supplements in the form of Ketovite tablets and liquid are standard practice.
- Nasogastric or gastrostomy feeding may be required.
- Regular skinfold thickness measurements and bone age assessments are helpful.

Clinical paediatrics for postgraduate exams

Renal osteodystrophy

Failure to hydroxylate vitamin D to its active form develops with progressive reduction in renal function, leading to decreased absorption of calcium and hyperphosphataemia, with the development of secondary hyperparathyroidism. Phosphate restriction is necessary by limiting the intake of milk products, phosphate binding with calcium carbonate and giving activated vitamin D supplementation.

Electrolyte balance

Salt supplementation and free water intake are essential in some children where underlying renal disease causes loss of salt and water. Bicarbonate supplements may be necessary to correct the acidosis.

Anaemia

Children generally show a normochromic normocytic anaemia. The rate of red cell production and life span are reduced. In addition to low levels of erythropoietin, poor dietary intake of iron and folate is also common and supplements may be necessary. Human recombinant erythropoietin injections are required but inhibitors may develop.

Hormone abnormalities

Poor growth is a common problem in CRF which results from growth hormone resistance with normal or high growth hormone levels. Trials to establish the efficacy and safety of human recombinant growth hormone replacement are currently underway. Pubertal delay with a poor pubertal growth spurt is also frequently encountered.

Dialysis and transplantation

Indications for transplant are:

● symptoms of increasing ECF expansion – hypertension and pulmonary oedema not responding to medical therapy
● end-stage deterioration in renal function.

Ideally, children are transplanted before dialysis is required, but occasionally a period of dialysis is necessary and may be either of the following:

Peritoneal dialysis
● Overnight cycling
● Continuous ambulatory peritoneal dialysis, with manual exchanges every 24 hours
● Preferable to haemodialysis as can be done by parents at home with less disruption to family and education.

Haemodialysis   Requires dialysis approximately three times per week, in hospital for up to 4 hours at a time.

Transplantation   This is always the aim when children develop end-stage CRF. Renal replacement programmes can be entered for all children with end-stage renal failure, although most centres choose 10 kg as a lower limit due to the difficulties of a very small child.

There are two types of transplant:

● cadaveric
● living-related donor – parent offers the best chance of success.

Transplantation necessitates lifelong immunosuppression with ciclosporin, prednisolone or azathioprine, which are not without significant unwanted side-effects. Success is generally good and graft rejection decreases with time. First-year graft survival is about 90%, reducing to 75–80% by 5 years.

COMMON SHORT CASES

The abdomen is an integral part of the clinical short cases and, as with a developmental assessment, a candidate should expect to be asked to perform this examination. However, in our opinion this is a chance to shine. There is a limited number of physical signs to be elicited, which have a limited number of possible causes.

HEPATOMEGALY, SPLENOMEGALY AND HEPATOSPLENOMEGALY

See Table 5.3, which is not intended to be an exhaustive list of conditions that may be met in the exam, but provides a framework within which the correct diagnosis may be sought. Candidates must know common causes of an enlarged liver and be able to search for associated signs to support their diagnosis, e.g. if you suspect right heart failure then offer to examine the cardiovascular system, or if you suspect infectious mononucleosis then ask the child for a history of a sore throat. Similarly, causes of mild, moderate and gross enlargement of the spleen should be well rehearsed and confirmatory signs looked for. It will usually be necessary to comment on the presence or absence of jaundice.

CHRONIC LIVER DISEASE

This is a common short case. Signs to look for should include:

- degree of jaundice (colour of skin)
- presence of portal hypertension (cardinal sign is splenomegaly)
- spider naevi (number and distribution)
- colour of stool
- evidence of pruritus
- obvious chest disease (cystic fibrosis)
- Kayser–Fleischer rings, best seen with a slit lamp and present in Wilson's disease
- surgical scar in the region of the liver would suggest a liver biopsy
- cirrhosis or a Kasai procedure or modification for extrahepatic biliary atresia.

ENLARGED KIDNEY(S)

- *Unilateral enlargement* – either hydronephrosis or possibly a cyst. The major differential is a Wilms' tumour which is very unlikely in the exam. Are you certain that enlargement is not bilateral?
- *Bilateral enlargement* – polycystic kidney disease or bilateral hydronephrosis.
- Check the back for spina bifida, and offer to check the blood pressure.

Table 5.3 Causes of hepatomegaly, *hepatosplenomegaly* and **splenomegaly**

Age group	Infection	Haematological	Metabolic/miscellaneous	Gastrointestinal	Cardiac	Malignant
Neonate	Congenital infections: Cytomegalovirus (++) Rubella (++) Toxoplasmosis (++)	Haemolytic disease of newborn (+)	Galactosaemia (++)	Neonatal hepatitis syndrome (+++) (including biliary atresia syndrome)	Heart failure (+++)	*Leukaemia* (+) *Lymphoma* (+) Neuroblastoma
Infancy and early childhood	Viral: Cytomegalovirus (++) Hepatitis (++) Epstein–Barr (+++) virus Bacterial: Septicaemia (+) **Subacute bacterial endocarditis (SBE)** (++) Protozoal: **Malaria** (++)	Sickle cell disease (++) **Sickle cell disease (young child)** (++) *Thalassaemia* (+++) **Spherocytosis** (+++)	Glycogen storage disorders (+++) (usually marked hepatomegaly) *Mucopolysaccharidoses* (+++) Reye's syndrome (++) *α-1-antitrypsin deficiency* (++)	**Portal hypertension** (+++)	Heart failure (+++)	*Leukaemia* (+) *Lymphoma* (+)
Older childhood and adolescence	As above and: **Malaria** (++) **Subacute bacterial endocarditis (SBE)** (++)	**Spherocytosis** (+++)	As above (except Reye's syndrome) and Wilson's disease (++) Juvenile chronic arthritis (++) Systemic lupus erythematosus (++)	**Portal hypertension** (+++)	Heart failure (+++)	*Leukaemia* (+) *Lymphoma* (+)

Seen in MRCP exam: (+++) commonly, (++) uncommonly, (+) rarely
Sections in: plain Roman type, hepatomegaly; italic type, hepatosplenomegaly; bold type, splenomegaly

CHRONIC RENAL FAILURE

- Look for evidence of peritoneal dialysis or vascular access.
- There may be evidence of anaemia and thrombocytopenia (petechial rash), suggesting the diagnosis of haemolytic uraemic syndrome, or there may be evidence of a previous (failed) renal transplant.
- Comment on the state of hydration of the patient, looking carefully for signs of fluid overload (sacral and periorbital oedema, raised jugular venous pressure), and check the weight chart at the end of the bed. Offer to check the blood pressure.

ABDOMINAL MASSES

- Chronic constipation, possibly Hirschsprung's disease
- Ectopic or transplanted kidney
- Palpable bladder – look for spinal lesion
- Intussusception and pyloric stenosis are very unlikely
- Malignancy is very unlikely in the exam.

SUMMARY OF ABDOMINAL EXAMINATION

INSPECTION
Expose the patient from the nipples to the knees

General
Dysmorphism, nutritional status, hair, jaundice, gastrostomy tubes, TPN lines, wearing nappies, scratch marks, spider naevi, bruising, race

Hands
Clubbing, pallor, xanthoma, leuconychia, koilonychia, palmar erythema

Face
Jaundice, pallor

Mouth
Pigmentation on lips, ulcers, dental caries, gum hypertrophy, macroglossia, cheilitis

Abdomen
Distension (5 Fs) – fat, faeces, fluid, flatus, fetus
Scars – incl. renal, herniae, biopsy scars
Visible organomegaly, caput medusa (veins drain away from umbilicus), distended abdominal veins
Hernia including umbilical (commoner in Afro-Caribbeans, Down's, MPS, hypothyroidism)
Genitalia, hydrocele
Nappy – stool colour, urine

PALPATION
Neck
Lymphadenopathy

Abdomen
Do not take your eyes off the child's face
Superficial and deep palpation in each of the quadrants
Hepatomegaly – size (use tape measure, not 'finger breadths'), smooth, tender, pulsatile (AV malformation), expansile (tricuspid regurgitation), splenomegaly, kidneys
Know how to explain the difference between liver, spleen and kidneys

PERCUSSION
Upper and lower borders of the liver, and spleen if enlarged
Ascites

AUSCULTATION
Bowel sounds, renal bruits (hypertension, neurofibromatosis)

ANYTHING ELSE?
Offer to examine the genitalia and also the anus for fistulae or skin tags
Plot height and weight on a growth chart appropriate for age and sex
Offer to inspect the stools and test the urine

Growth and endocrinology

6

Assessment of growth parameters, height, weight and head circumference is an integral part of examining children, although you will rarely be asked to do this in the exam. A detailed understanding of growth charts (both distance and velocity) is important, as is the ability to work out decimal age and calculate height velocity. A comprehensive explanation of these techniques is available on the Tanner and Whitehouse growth charts and the newer Child Growth Foundation charts. Clinical examination of the endocrine system is largely confined to examination of the thyroid gland and the staging of puberty. You should be knowledgeable about and able to recognize syndromes associated with disorders of growth (e.g. Turner's syndrome and Russell–Silver syndrome, which are discussed in more detail in Ch. 11).

GROWTH

The growth of a child and final height potential are dependent on a number of endogenous and exogenous factors (Table 6.1). Consequently the diagnosis of the child who is short and growing slowly comprises the whole of paediatrics and is not just confined to endocrine disorders. Short stature is arbitrarily defined as height below a given centile for age and sex. This was generally taken as the third centile, but community growth charts mark the 0.4th and second centiles, although only 1 in 250 children below the 0.4th centile will be normal in growth terms. The rate of growth (height velocity) is a much better guide to whether growth is normal than a simple height measurement. In this chapter we discuss the clinical approach to the child who is short, in order to distinguish those children who are normal from those with underlying pathology who require treatment. Some of the easily recognizable syndromes are discussed in detail in Chapter 11.

HISTORY

Birth history
- Antenatal/maternal problems
- Gestation
- Birthweight/length
- Neonatal problems.

A child who suffered from prolonged intrauterine growth retardation (IUGR) is unlikely, despite 'catch-up' growth, to achieve full growth potential, but nevertheless will grow at a *normal* rate.

PMH   Chronic illness.
Drug history   Long-term steroids.
Dietary history

Table 6.1 Factors influencing growth

Familial Biological parental short stature	*Endocrine disorders* Hypothalamus – true precocious puberty
Congenital conditions Skeletal dysplasias Chromosomal disorders, e.g. Turner's syndrome IUGR	Pituitary – growth hormone deficiency Target organs – hypothyroidism, Cushing's Target tissues – Laron type 'dwarfism' IGF interactions – reduced IGF-1 response
Constitutional delay of growth and puberty	*Environmental/psychological* Nutritional – malnutrition
Chronic systemic disorders Respiratory – asthma, cystic fibrosis Cardiovascular – congenital heart disease Gastrointestinal – IBD, coeliac disease Renal – chronic renal failure	Socioeconomic – poverty Psychosocial deprivation

Family history – including age at onset of puberty
Social history
Systems enquiry

EXAMINATION

Age
Convert to decimal age to enable an accurate plot on the growth chart.

Height

Child sitting and standing   Look for evidence of disproportion (either short legs or short trunk in relation to standing height). The best method is to measure sitting height and calculate sub-ischial leg length (which is standing height less sitting height). Using the appropriate Tanner and Whitehouse chart, the sitting height and sub-ischial leg length can be plotted for the patient's age and should, if there is no significant disproportion, fall on similar centiles.

Adult height potential (Child Growth Foundation 1996)

Female   Calculate the adult height potential of a girl as follows:

$$\text{Mid-parental height (MPH, cm)} = \frac{\text{(father's height + mother's height)}}{2} - 7$$

Male   The adult height potential of a boy is calculated as follows:

$$\text{Mid-parental height (MPH, cm)} = \frac{\text{(father's height + mother's height)}}{2} + 7$$

Mid-parental centile   Plot the child's adult height potential on the chart and the nearest centile line is the 50th centile, known as the mid-parental centile (MPC).

Target centile range   The child's curve would be expected to follow a centile somewhere between the ninth and 91st centiles (mid-parental height +/– 8.5cm), known as the target centile range (TCR).

Nutritional status
● Weight
● Skinfold thickness – if a pair of calipers is available.

Pubertal status

Signs of dysmorphic features

Signs of chronic disease

CLASSIFICATION

In the light of the above information you should now be able to classify the child into one of the following four groups:

A dysmorphic child with a recognizable syndrome   For example:

● Turner's syndrome in female
● Down's syndrome
● Noonan's syndrome
● Russell–Silver syndrome
● Prader–Willi syndrome.

Disproportionate short stature   A skeletal survey will usually be required for diagnosis.

● Short back and limbs, e.g.
    — spondyloepiphyseal dysplasias
    — mucopolysaccharidoses
    — metatrophic dwarfism
● Short limbs, e.g.
    — achondroplasia
    — hypochondroplasia
    — metaphyseal chondroplasia.

Short but thin   Search for associated chronic disease, e.g.:

● cardiovascular disease
● respiratory (cystic fibrosis)
● malabsorption (coeliac)
● chronic inflammatory bowel disease
● renal (chronic renal failure).

Also consider:

● psychosocial deprivation
● anorexia nervosa.

Short and fat (with increased subcutaneous fat)   This would suggest an endocrine cause, e.g.:

● panhypopituitarism
● isolated growth hormone deficiency
● hypothyroidism
● pseudohypoparathyroidism
● Cushing's syndrome.

Figure 6.1 presents an algorithm for the assessment of a child with short stature.

DISCUSSION POINTS

Indications for growth hormone therapy

The decision to commence growth hormone (GH) therapy should only be made by a specialist paediatric endocrinologist and should be based on the child's need for treatment rather than the parents' demands.

Growth hormone deficiency

Turner's syndrome Growth hormone replacement in these girls has been widely studied. Meta-analysis of the results of large cohorts of patients in multicentre and multinational studies has shown that GH increases height

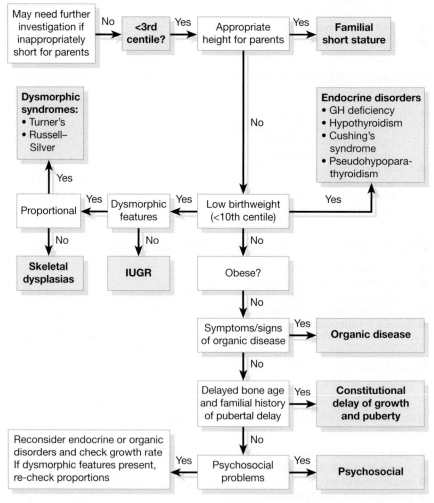

Fig. 6.1 Algorithm for the diagnosis of short stature. (Courtesy of Serono Laboratories.)

Clinical paediatrics for postgraduate exams

in Turner's syndrome, with many now surpassing 159 cm, which is within the normal adult range. The gain in height is positively correlated to the dose and most of the gain is achieved within the first 3 years of therapy. Oxandrolone in conjunction with GH improves final height and achieves it at a faster rate, thus reducing the time on GH. There is no evidence to support the use of oestrogen to improve final height.

Renal failure   Growth hormone is effective in improving growth in patients with chronic renal failure, on dialysis, or post-transplant.

Down's syndrome   Although not routinely used, GH has been shown to maintain a normal height velocity, which decreases on stopping treatment. There are concerns about using GH in conditions with chromosome fragility, as this may be associated with an increased risk of leukaemia.

Juvenile chronic arthritis   Preliminary studies suggest that GH may partially counteract the adverse effects of glucocorticoids on growth and metabolism in patients with chronic inflammatory disease.

Idiopathic short stature   Short-term administration of GH to children with idiopathic short stature results in an increase in growth rate. Recent results from studies of long-term administration of GH have shown that adult height can only marginally be above the predicted adult height. There is significant psychological disadvantage from short stature and improvement with GH therapy has not been demonstrated in studies, but some individuals could benefit.

Management of constitutional delay of growth and puberty
Delayed puberty is defined arbitrarily as no evidence of puberty by age 13 in girls and 14 in boys. The majority of these children have no endocrine abnormality, and their pubertal development and growth spurt are simply consequences of primary delay (constitutional delay of growth and puberty). Short stature and lack of sexual development can result in psychological upset, which may persist even when fully developed. Although controversial, research has suggested that a delay in the 'tempo' of pubertal maturation may interfere with normal bone accretion occurring during puberty, with consequent osteoporosis in later life. This would suggest that intervention may be neceessary not only for emotional and social reasons but also to optimize bone mass accretion. The treatment should not interfere with final height prognosis and must be safe. There is good evidence that oxandrolone (an anabolic steroid), when given in a dose of 2.5 mg daily for 3 months in early established puberty, will advance the growth rate of boys without detriment to final height.

PUBERTAL STAGING

The ability to stage puberty accurately is important in clinical practice and may be required in the long case (Figs 6.2 and 6.3). It is the loss of the normal harmony of puberty which implies an endocrinopathy, e.g. the presence of pubic and axillary hair in a girl without breast development, characteristic of congenital adrenal hyperplasia or Turner's syndrome.

The criteria below are as described in *Growth at Adolescence* by J M Tanner (Blackwell, Oxford, 1962).

Female breast changes	Male genital stages
BI Prepubertal	GI Preadolescent
BII Breast bud	GII Enlargement, change in texture
BIII Juvenile smooth contour	GIII Growth in length and circumference
BIV Areola and papilla project above breast	GIV Further development of glans penis, darkening of scrotal skin
BV Adult	GV Adult genitalia

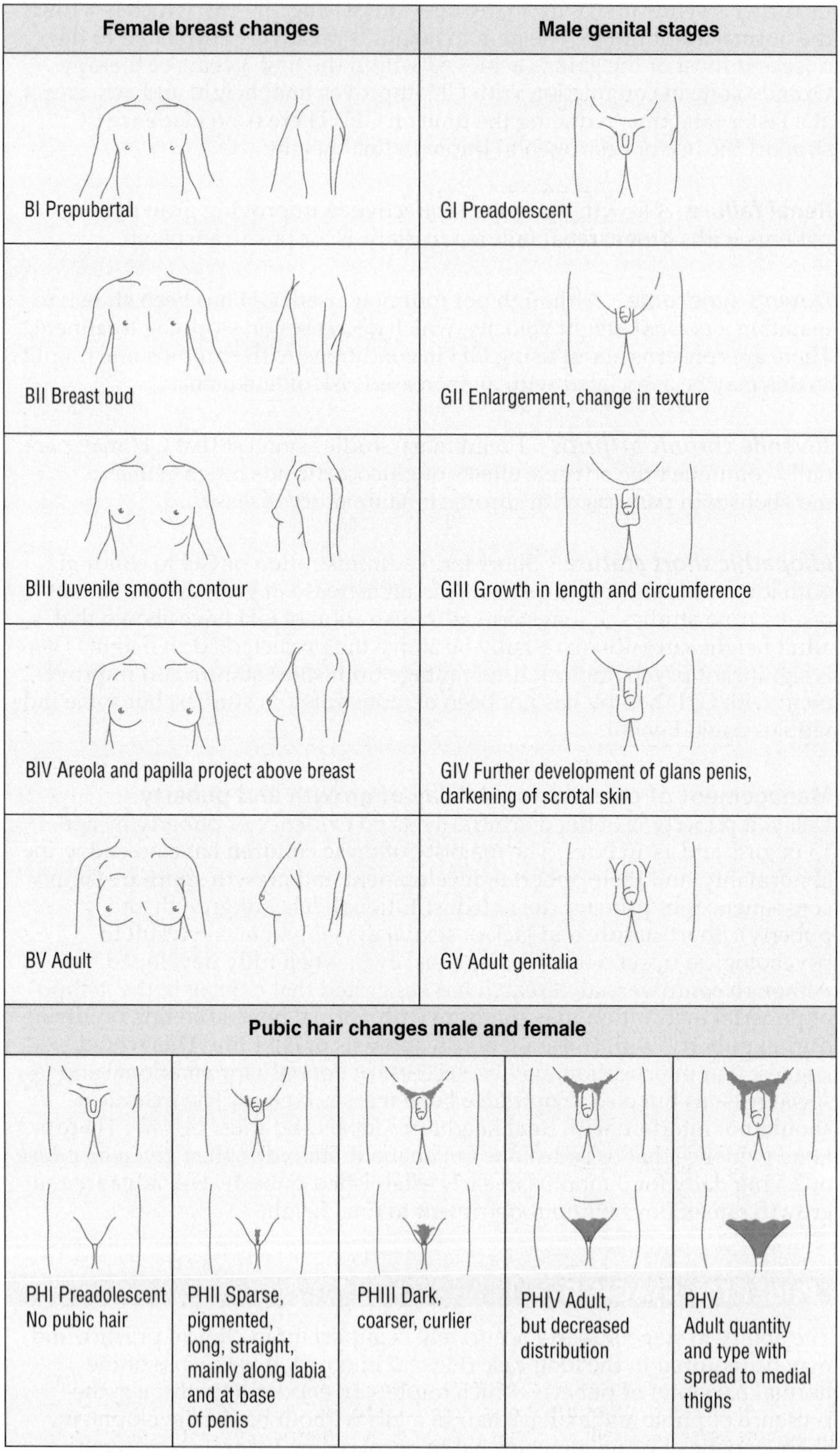

Pubic hair changes male and female

PHI Preadolescent No pubic hair	PHII Sparse, pigmented, long, straight, mainly along labia and at base of penis	PHIII Dark, coarser, curlier	PHIV Adult, but decreased distribution	PHV Adult quantity and type with spread to medial thighs

Fig. 6.2 Schematic drawings of male and female stages of puberty, as described by Tanner.

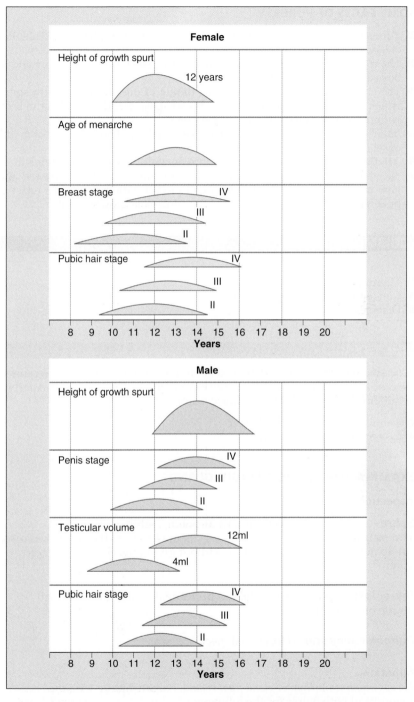

Fig. 6.3 Schematic representation of the timing of pubertal changes in males and females. Pubertal changes are shown according to the Tanner stages of puberty. (Diagrams based on Zitelli B J, Davis H W Atlas of Pediatric Physical Diagnosis, 2nd edn, Lippincott, Philadelphia, 1992 and Johnson T R, Moore W M, Jeffries J E Children are Different, 2nd edn, Ross Laboratories, Division of Abbot Laboratories, Columbus, OH, 1978.)

Clinical paediatrics for postgraduate exams

SOME FACTS OF PUBERTY

- Puberty usually begins with breast development in girls and testicular enlargement in boys.
- The mean age at onset of puberty in girls (breast stage 2) is 11 years and in boys (4 mL testicular volume) is 11.2 years.
- The characteristic difference is in the timing of onset of the growth spurt, which occurs early in girls, between breast stages 2 and 3, and later in boys with the acquisition of 10 mL volume testes.
- In girls, the attainment of breast stage 4 is usually, but not always, before the onset of menstruation.
- After the onset of menarche, only approximately 5 cm of growth remain.
- Skeletal maturity is a good guide as to how much growth has passed and how much is left to come, but it cannot predict with certainty the onset of puberty or the timing of the peak of the adolescent growth spurt.

COMMON LONG CASES

- Thyroid disorders
- Congenital adrenal hyperplasia
- Diabetes

THE THYROID

Assessment of the thyroid gland can be divided into two parts and requires the candidate to listen carefully to the examiner's instructions, particularly in the short case section of the clinical exam:

- examination of the thyroid gland
- assessment of thyroid status.

EXAMINATION OF THE THYROID GLAND

Inspection

Goitre   Asking the child to sit with the chin slightly elevated may demonstrate a goitre. A goitre can be seen to elevate as the child swallows, but do not specifically test for this without giving the child a drink of water.

Thyroglossal cyst   Ask the child to protrude the tongue – a cyst will elevate on doing this.

Thyroidectomy scar   Horizontal 'necklace' scar.

Palpation
Always examine the thyroid gland from behind. Palpate lightly with the fingertips of both hands for the following:

- define the upper and lower borders of the lateral lobes
- consistency of the gland
- thyroglossal cysts are situated in the midline and tend to be fluctuant

- movement of the gland
  - confirm that the gland, which is attached to the pretracheal fascia, moves when the child swallows some water
  - a thyroglossal cyst moves upwards on protrusion of the tongue
- retrosternal extension and tracheal deviation should be examined for by palpating in the suprasternal notch
- enlarged cervical lymph glands.

Auscultation
Systolic bruit may accompany a diffuse toxic goitre.

ASSESSMENT OF THYROID STATUS

A child with a goitre may be hyperthyroid, hypothyroid or euthyroid.

Hypothyroidism
The most common cause of this is autoimmune thyroiditis, which is more prevalent in girls and is a common short case in the exams, often with a goitre. Clinical features are obtained from history and examination.

History
- Slow growth and pubertal delay
- Cold intolerance
- Poor concentration/deterioration in school work
- Learning difficulties
- Constipation.

Examination
- General
  - short stature (may be antedated by subnormal height velocity)
  - delayed puberty (but occasionally may be advanced)
  - obesity
  - slow speech, thought and movement
- Face
  - pale, puffy eyes with loss of eyebrows
  - thin dry hair
  - dry skin
- Pulse – bradycardia (plus decreased pulse pressure)
- Hands – cold peripheries
- Reflexes – delayed relaxation.

Hyperthyroidism
Graves' disease is the most common cause of thyrotoxicosis and is three times more common in females than in males. Clinical features are obtained from history and examination.

History
- Anxiety, restlessness
- Sweating
- Thin, weight loss
- Increased appetite
- Rapid growth in height (with concomitant advancement in bone age)

- Heat intolerance
- Learning difficulties/behavioural problems.

Examination
- General – hyperpigmentation, vitiligo and very rarely pretibial myxoedema
- Hands
  — fine tremor
  — warm and sweaty
  — tachycardia
- Neck – goitre (bruit)
- Eye signs (not always present)
  — exophthalmos
  — lid retraction: the eyelid fails to bisect a cord across the iris and therefore the sclerae are visible above the iris
  — lid lag: ask the child to follow the movements of your finger slowly upwards and downwards. The sclera becomes visible above the iris on downward gaze as the eyelid is slow to follow the movement of the eye
  — rarely external ophthalmoplegia involving lateral or superior rectus muscles
- Cardiovascular
  — hyperactive praecordium and there may be an ejection systolic murmur
  — blood pressure is elevated, with an increased pulse pressure
- Neurological – proximal muscle weakness.

CONGENITAL ADRENAL HYPERPLASIA

Congenital adrenal hyperplasia (CAH) is an autosomal recessive disorder, occurring in 1 in 10 000 births, with more than 90% of cases due to a deficiency of the 21-hydroxylase enzyme required for cortisol biosynthesis, and 5% of cases being associated with a deficiency of the 11-β-hydroxylase enzyme. The clinical hallmark of the disease is virilization due to lack of negative feedback on adrenocorticotrophic hormone (ACTH) causing excess adrenal androgen production. About two-thirds of patients with 21-hydroxylase deficiency are salt-losers (i.e. one-third are non-salt-losers and can present later).

HISTORY

Presentation

Ambiguous genitalia   The female child usually presents with virilization of the external genitalia at birth. The degree of virilization may be pronounced such that the child may masquerade as a cryptorchid male with or without hypospadias. Inappropriate gender assignment has tragic consequences, and in the newborn baby with ambiguous genitalia this should not be attempted until the results of appropriate investigations are known.

Salt-losing crisis   A male infant with CAH rarely has signs of virilization, and the presentation is commonly in the second or third week of life with a salt-losing crisis. About two-thirds of children are salt-losers.

Tall stature/precocious puberty   Males with CAH who are not salt-losers present in childhood with signs of virilization and increased linear growth. The testes remain prepubertal in size, indicating that the source of androgen production is adrenal not testicular.

Medical treatment

Steroid replacement for life   Glucocorticoid replacement +/− mineralocorticoid – the cortisol secretion rate is about 12 mg/m^2 per day. Glucocorticoid therapy is usually with hydrocortisone (10–15 mg/m^2 per day) in two or three divided doses with 50% of the daily dose in the morning. Mineralocorticoid therapy is with fludrocortisone (0.05–0.1 mg daily) if there is salt loss. Mineralocorticoid replacement therapy should be sufficient to maintain plasma renin activity within the appropriate range for age. Infants may require additional sodium chloride supplementation.

Surgical management
This depends on the degree of virilization of the external genitalia.

- Cliteroplasty with reduction in the size of the enlarged clitoris is usually performed in infancy.
- Vaginoplasty, with division of the fused labial folds if required, is delayed until puberty.

Family history
A careful family history may reveal a history of previous unexplained male infant deaths.

Intercurrent illness/hospital admissions
- Are the parents aware of the need for additional steroid replacement during illness or surgery?
- Has the child required admission to hospital for i.v. steroid administration due to illness?

Home monitoring
17-OH-progesterone can be measured in saliva or from paper blood spots, and serial samples can be collected from the patient, once out of nappies, at home by the parent and subsequently analysed. These intermittent daily profiles are extremely useful in the biochemical assessment of control.

EXAMINATION

Genitalia

Female
- Cliteromegaly – although the patient may already have undergone cliteroplasty
- Fused labial folds – unlikely to have undergone vaginoplasty as yet.

Male
- Usually entirely normal
- May be virilized if presenting with precocious puberty, but will have normal-sized testes.

Blood pressure
Hypertension.

- Hallmark of 11-β-hydroxylase deficiency
- May be iatrogenic due to overtreatment.

Growth
- Children may present with tall stature
- Indicator of overtreatment – growth velocity and bone age are used to assess the degree of control
- Bone age estimation provides useful information about final height prognosis and degree of adrenal androgen suppression but is particularly unreliable during infancy when satisfactory control is necessary for normal growth.

Weight/striae
Weight gain, striae and hypertension are indicators of hypercortisolism.

INVESTIGATIONS

CAH is the commonest cause of ambiguous genitalia in the newborn, but a karyoptye is essential to exclude under-virilization of the male due to androgen insensitivity syndrome or androgen biosynthetic defects. You must be familiar with the investigations required to elucidate the cause of ambiguous genitalia in the newborn infant.

Karyotype
- Over-virilized female
- Under-virilized male.

Pelvic ultasound scan To look for the presence of a uterus and gonads.

Biochemistry Electrolytes will be normal at birth even in salt-losers, and they thus require regular measurement.

24-hour urinary steroid profile Elevated plasma 17-OH progesterone is indicative of CAH, but do not measure on day 1 as 17-OH will be high anyway due to stress response or if the child is premature.

DISCUSSION POINTS

Prenatal diagnosis and treatment
Timely diagnosis of this condition is important, since infants may suffer adrenal insufficiency, which carries a high mortality rate. The measurement of 17-OH-progesterone in amniotic fluid is a reliable test for the prenatal diagnosis of 21-hydroxylase deficiency. However, this is too late to attempt to prevent virilization of a female fetus by the maternal administration of dexamethasone. Chorionic villus biopsy would allow earlier prenatal diagnosis, but current DNA probes for the 21-hydroxylase gene are not yet able to detect all patients with CAH. Some groups have treated mothers with 'at risk' pregnancies with dexamethasone from 5 weeks' gestation until 10 days before amniocentesis; if the fetus is female and the levels of

17-OH-progesterone are elevated then dexamethasone can be recommended. The results suggest that there is a reduction in virilization of the external genitalia.

Newborn screening

The incidence of CAH is low (1 in 10 000 Caucasian births) and the measurement of 17-OH-progesterone in a filter paper blood spot is technically simple, although false-positive results may occur in sick preterm infants. Routine screening would be expected to avoid problems such as salt-losing crises and inappropriate gender assignment, although this is not standard practice in the UK at present.

CAH is not the only cause of ambiguous genitalia and you must be aware of other underlying causes. Female pseudohermaphroditism (46XX) describes virilization of external genitalia and normal ovaries and Müllerian structures. This may be a consequence of excessive fetal androgen production (CAH, as decribed above) or exposure to increased transplacental androgen (maternal or iatrogenic), or it may be idiopathic. Male pseudohermaphroditism (46XY) describes incomplete virilization of external genitalia and normally differentiated testes. This may be due to abnormal secretion or action of Müllerian inhibitory factor (MIH) – persistent Müllerian duct syndrome, impaired Leydig cell activity or impaired peripheral tissue androgen metabolism. Rarely it is associated with dysmorphic syndromes, e.g. Smith–Lemli–Opitz.

The infant may have isolated cliteromegaly or more pronounced virilization with partial or complete fusion of the labioscrotal folds. The most important aspect of the clinical examination is to look for the presence of gonads. If no gonads are present, the most likely diagnosis is CAH due to 21-hydroxylase deficiency in a genotypic female. Male pseudohermaphroditism with intra-abdominal testes is much less common and true hermaphroditism is very rare. If one gonad is palpable, mixed gonadal dysgenesis (usually with XO/XY karyotype) is least uncommon. Two palpable gonads are most likely due to male pseudohermaphroditism. Human chorionic gonadotrophin (HCG) testing to measure testosterone, dihydrotestosterone, dihydroepianprosterone and androstenedione will help to distinguish between 5-alpha-reductase deficiency, testosterone biosynthetic disorders and androgen receptor or postreceptor defects. Genitograms may be helpful in imaging the internal genitalia and lower urinary tract.

Sex of rearing is made jointly between the parents, surgeon and paediatric endocrinologist. This decision will be based upon the appearance of the external genitalia and functional possibilities in the context of information (cytogenetic, biochemical and radiological) about the nature of the underlying defect and the implications for development at puberty.

DIABETES MELLITUS

Children with diabetes mellitus (DM) are readily available for paediatric postgraduate exams. Establish a good rapport and *listen* to what the child is telling you.

Definition The detection of a raised blood sugar level in the presence of glycosuria and ketonuria is pathognomonic of DM and diagnosis rarely requires glucose tolerance testing. The WHO has defined blood glucose concentrations to aid diagnosis: fasting blood glucose >6.7 mmol/L and 2-hour post-glucose load (1.75 g/kg) of >10 mmol/L.

HISTORY

We suggest that in your clinical approach to a patient with diabetes you include the following areas.

Review the history and presentation

Symptoms pre-diagnosis
- Length of symptoms
- Polyuria/polydipsia/weight loss
- ?Delay in diagnosis/conflict with medical staff.

Clinical condition at diagnosis
- Well
- Unwell with ketosis.

Initial management
- Well – hospital stay/outpatient
- Unwell – diabetic ketoacidosis: admitted to high dependency?

Duration of HDU/ward stay
What was the patient's initial reaction to:
- the diagnosis
- injections
- glucose monitoring
- diet?

How was the education package delivered?
Were the family well supported by the diabetic liaison nurses?

Subsequent management

Insulin
- Free mixing with syringes
- Pens.

Monitoring
- Blood glucose
  — frequency
  — timing
  — who checks it?
  — recorded in diary?
- Types of meter

Diet
- Timing of food
  — regular meals three times per day
  — regular snacks × 2–3 (including supper) per day
- Content of food – healthy diet
  — complex carbohydrates
  — low fat.

Assessing control

Aim for blood glucose
- Majority of pre-meal readings: 4–10 mmol/L
- Avoid hypoglycaemia.

HbA1c: 7–8.5% Measurement of glycosylated haemoglobin is important in the assessment of control as it gives a measure of overall blood sugar control over the previous 6 weeks.

School history
It is clearly important to establish whether attendance or performance at school has been compromised by the condition. The requirement for daily injections may be a source of bullying and teasing.

Family history
- Father with DM – 7% risk to child
- Mother with DM – 5% risk to child
- Sibling with DM – 5% risk to another sibling.

Psychosocial aspects
Assess the impact of this disease on the child, parents and siblings. Establish any areas of difficulty, e.g.:

- injections
- glucose monitoring
- diet adherence
- omitting insulin
- teasing at school
- anxiety, e.g. concerning hypoglycaemic episodes during both day and night
- support at school
- independence
  — staying over with friends
  — going away with school to camp
- adolescence – fabrication of test results and rejection of authoritarian management are common, particularly during adolescence.

Level of knowledge about management of diabetes
This is not an opportunity for the candidate to educate the family.

Complications
These are very rare in childhood/adolescence.

EXAMINATION
- Height and weight must be plotted on a growth chart including pubertal staging.
- Injection sites – lipohypertrophy is very common.
- Long-term complications of DM are very unlikely in children. Nevertheless you should examine for the following:
  — optic fundus for retinopathy
  — sensory neuropathy
  — blood pressure
    — hypertension
    — postural hypotension may be indicative of an autonomic neuropathy
    — urinalysis – protein: the presence of persistent proteinuria is generally agreed to herald the onset of nephropathy. Permanent microalbuminuria has been shown to predict clinical nephropathy within 10 years in insulin-dependent DM.

DISCUSSION POINTS

There are many possible avenues of discussion and, because DM is common, the candidate would be expected to have a broad knowledge of the subject. Some common issues are briefly outlined below.

Clinical management

There is an increasing move away from spending prolonged periods of time in hospital at diagnosis, if clinically well, towards managing this condition by the multidisciplinary team in the community. In many areas there are specialist liaison nurses who work closely with the hospital diabetic specialists, GP and dietician to support the child at the time of diagnosis and thereafter.

There is a wide range of insulin regimens, and insulin can be administered by:

- insulin syringe
- insulin pen device
- continuous subcutaneous insulin infusion.

Types of insulin

New rapid-acting analogues   Immediate onset and action over 2 hours, e.g.:
- Humalog
- Novorapid.

Short-acting soluble insulins   Inject 20–30 minutes before a meal and action lasts over 4 hours.

Long-acting insulins
- Gradual increase in insulin
- Works over 8–12 hours.

Regimens

Twice daily   Combination of short- and long-acting; either of:
- free mix with syringe
- pre-mixed via pen.

Basal bolus   One of the following:
- fast-acting pre-meal and long-acting overnight
- very fast-acting with small amount of long-acting in the morning
- very fast-acting pre-meals and snacks with long-acting overnight.

Combination of twice daily and basal bolus

Continuous infusion via pump with very fast-acting analogues   Delivery of basal rate and can administer meal boluses.

Doses   The conventional insulin requirement is 0.7–1.0 U/kg per day in early childhood, increasing to 1–1.5 U/kg per day with the pubertal growth spurt. Newly diagnosed patients with some endogenous production of insulin will require significantly less ('honeymoon' period).

Basal bolus/pump
- 50% as fast-acting and 50% as long-acting.

Twice-daily injections
- Two-thirds of daily dose in the morning pre-breakfast
- One-third of daily dose in the evening pre-evening meal
  — one-third of dose as fast-acting
  — two-thirds as long-acting.

Specific situations **Somogyi effect** – asymptomatic hypoglycaemia in the middle of the night activates counter-regulatory hormones to drive up blood glucose, resulting in morning hyperglycaemia. In this situation, the urge to increase the insulin dosage should be resisted until the result of a night-time blood sugar profile is known (i.e. if there is morning hyperglycaemia, exclude nocturnal hypoglycaemia).

Relevance of the Diabetes Control and Complications Trial (DCCT) related to paediatrics

The single most important relevant message from the DCCT for children is that young people with diabetes and their families can work together in partnership with the support of a variety of health care professionals towards the shared aim of improving control in the context of improved quality of life. The key is avoiding tight glycaemic control whilst avoiding severe or recurrent hypoglycaemia (particularly in young children) in the context of normal growth and psychological development.

Future prospects for treatment

Pancreatic and islet cell transplantation have been explored in DM but, due to autoimmunity and the shortage of available islet tissue, remain experimental. Externally worn pumps delivering subcutaneous insulin are increasingly being used in children, although they are not yet widely used in the UK. Immunosuppressive regimens designed to curtail the process of beta-cell destruction have been employed with some success after diagnosis. However, the potential renal toxicity of ciclosporin probably precludes its use at the present time.

COMMON SHORT CASES

- Thyrotoxicosis
- Hypothyroidism
- Precocious puberty
- Pseudohypoparathyroidism
- Tall stature
  - Marfan's syndrome
  - homocystinuria
  - Klinefelter's syndrome
  - Soto's syndrome.

THYROTOXICOSIS

- Graves' disease is the most common cause of thyrotoxicosis and occurs pre-dominantly in females (at least 3:1).
- There is an increased incidence in Down's syndrome, diabetes mellitus and Addison's disease and there is commonly a family history of thyroid disease.
- See page 114 for examination findings.

HYPOTHYROIDISM IN THE PRESENCE OF A GOITRE

- The most common cause is autoimmune thyroiditis, which is more common in girls.
- Examination findings are described earlier in the chapter (p. 113).

Growth and endocrinology

PRECOCIOUS PUBERTY

Definition   The acquisition of secondary sexual characteristics before the age of 8 years in girls and 9 years in boys. Early puberty is more common in girls but is more likely to have a pathological cause in boys. Conventionally, precocious puberty is considered to be either 'true' or 'pseudo' (Table 6.2).

True precocious puberty   This is the appearance of secondary sexual characteristics due to premature activation of the hypothalamic–pituitary–gonadal (HPG) axis. It may be physiological or pathological.

Pseudo-precocious puberty   The appearance of pubertal characteristics is not due to premature activation of the HPG axis. The source of sex hormones is the adrenal glands or gonads independent of pituitary gonadotrophin secretion. Rarely, extrapituitary gonadotrophin-secreting tumours may be the cause.

CLINICAL EXAMINATION IN GIRLS

The main differentiation is between pseudo-precocious puberty with androgenization alone (e.g. pubic and axillary hair, clitoromegaly) and true precocious puberty with oestrogenization and androgenization (but not clitoromegaly), (e.g. breast development, menstruation may occur, pubic and axillary hair).

The two important causes of pseudo-precocious puberty are:

● congenital adrenal hyperplasia (21-hydroxylase deficiency)
● virilizing adrenal tumour.

True precocious puberty is, in the majority of girls (about 90%), due to idiopathic premature activation of the HPG axis. Other causes include:

● CNS tumours
● hydrocephalus
● post-meningitis
● hypothyroidism
● specific syndromes, e.g. neurofibromatosis (Ch. 11), tuberous sclerosis (Ch. 11) and Albright's syndrome – a triad of true precocious puberty, polyostotic fibrous dysplasia of bones, and areas of skin pigmentation.

Table 6.2 Summary of common causes of precocious puberty

Boys	Girls
True precocious puberty	*True precocious puberty*
(testes >4 ml)	*(oestrogenization and androgenization)*
CNS tumour	Idiopathic (50%)
Idiopathic (50%)	
Pseudo-precocious puberty	*Psuedo-precocious puberty*
(testes <4 ml)	*(with androgenization and clitoromegaly)*
Congenital adrenal hyperplasia	Congenital adrenal hyperplasia
(21–hydroxylase deficiency)	(21–hydroxylase deficiency)
Adrenal virilizing tumour	Adrenal virilizing tumour

CLINICAL EXAMINATION IN BOYS

Precocious puberty in boys is uncommon and is likely to be pathological, particularly intracranial tumours. Testicular examination is often helpful.

If the testes are *prepubertal* (<4 mL) the diagnosis is suggestive of pseudo-precocious puberty due to extragonadal androgen secretion, e.g.:

● adrenal tumour
● adrenal hyperplasia.

In true precocious puberty, the testes are of *pubertal* volume (>4 mL) due to gonadotrophin secretion from the pituitary, e.g.:

● CNS tumour (pineal, hypothalamic, pituitary)
● hydrocephalus
● post-meningitis
● hypothyroidism
● specific syndromes (as for girls, but excluding Albright's syndrome)
● idiopathic premature activation of the HPG axis (about 50% of cases).

An exception to this rule of assessing testicular volumes to determine whether puberty is true or not is in the case of HCG-secreting tumours, which are more common in boys. Hepatoblastoma and teratoma may secrete gonadotrophins, which will cause enlargement of the testes and androgenization from Leydig cell stimulation.

SUMMARY OF THE EXAMINATION OF THE CHILD WITH EARLY PUBERTY

● Measure height, and assess growth rate if possible
● Accurate pubertal staging
● Palpate for a goitre and determine thyroid status
● Search for skin pigmentation or depigmentation and other signs of the neurocutaneous syndromes
● Careful examination of the central nervous system including fundoscopy and visual fields
● Abdominal palpation.

PSEUDOHYPOPARATHYROIDISM

Although this is an uncommon condition, it is commonly encountered in exams. The disorder is inherited in an autosomal dominant fashion with incomplete penetrance, although it is twice as common in females as it is in males. Its onset is in childhood with symptoms of hypocalcaemia, including tetany, muscle cramps and convulsions, resulting from renal tubular insensitivity to parathyroid hormone.

In type 1 (Albright's hereditary osteodystrophy) there is no phosphaturic response to PTH administration and a blunted urinary cyclic AMP increase. In type 2, the defect is beyond the cyclic AMP generation step so the cyclic AMP response to PTH is normal but the phosphaturic response is defective.

Characteristic features
● Short stature
● Obesity
● Round face and short neck

- Shortening of the fourth and fifth metacarpals
- Subcutaneous nodules
- Tooth enamel hypoplasia
- Mild learning difficulties
- Calcification of the basal ganglia.

TALL STATURE

It can be extremely difficult to recognize that patients are tall when they are lying or sitting down. If you suspect that they are tall begin your assessment by asking them to stand, and offer to measure them and plot the height on a distance chart. The clinical diagnostic problem is to establish if patients are tall in relation to their parents. Familial tall stature is the commonest problem in the clinic but Marfan's syndrome is more common in postgraduate exams.

Causes of tall stature

Familial
Associated with dysmorphic features
- Marfan's syndrome
- Homocystinuria
- Cerebral gigantism (Soto's syndrome)*
- Beckwith–Wiedemann syndrome*
- Klinefelter's syndrome.
  Endocrine disorders
- Pituitary gigantism
- Thyrotoxicosis*
- Precocious puberty*
- Adrenal disease – either congenital adrenal hyperplasia or functioning adrenal tumour.*

(* Final height not excessive.)

These disorders are described in more detail in *Paediatric Short Cases for Postgraduate Examinations* by A Thomson, H Wallace and T Stephenson (Churchill Livingstone, Edinburgh, 2003).

The nervous system

7

Candidates are often confounded by a simple request to 'look at this child's eyes' or 'examine this child's legs'. To deal with these commonplace clinical tasks, you must have a well rehearsed routine for examining each part of the nervous system. The neurological examination is the most difficult of the system examinations because it consists of many separate parts and because the neurological examination, as taught to medical students, presumes that the patient is fully cooperative. Much of this formal examination of the nervous system is possible with many children of school age and above, provided your instructions are simple; this is dealt with later in this chapter. However, far more difficult is the assessment of infants, toddlers or older handicapped children, in whom cooperation is minimal and observation of what they choose to do is more instructive than their compliance with actions which you have requested them to carry out.

It is important to understand the fundamental difference between the developmental and neurological assessments, although of course they are complementary and there will often be overlap. Developmental examination assesses the acquisition of learned skills, whereas the neurological examination assesses the integrity of the underlying nervous system and aims to make a neuroanatomical diagnosis of the site of any abnormality.

Examination of the nervous system can be divided up into the following parts:

- cranial nerves (pp. 125–143)
- examination of a baby/toddler (pp. 143–158)
- examination of an older child (pp. 158–167)
- examination of limb girdle and trunk (p. 167)
- examination of the cerebellar system (pp. 167–168)
- higher function (pp. 168–169).

You will not be expected to examine the whole nervous system of the child but may be asked some of the following:

- Can this child see?
- Can this child hear?
- Assess this child's gait.
- Examine this child's legs.
- This child has short stature. Would you like to examine his/her eyes?

CRANIAL NERVES

Before examining the cranial nerves, it is essential to ascertain quickly the child's level of understanding and ability to carry out simple instructions.

Table 7.1 Site of cranial nerve nuclei

Site	Cranial nerve nuclei
Midbrain	III
	IV
Pons	V
	VI
	VII
	VIII
Medulla	IX
	X
	XI
	XII

Asking a few simple questions at the start will also help to establish a rapport with the child, e.g. 'What is your teddy's name?' A detailed knowledge of neuroanatomy is not required for paediatric postgraduate exams and the information given here is not exhaustive. We wish to emphasize nerve functions which can be tested at the bedside and which are important in clinical paediatric neurology. However, one useful and simple guide to the pathology underlying a cranial nerve lesion is the site of the cranial nerve nuclei (Table 7.1).

I: OLFACTORY NERVE

Testing of smell is rarely required and should only be offered if:

● the child complains of loss of taste or smell
● the child has evidence of a visual field defect
● the child has had a frontal tumour or surgery.

Ask the child to shut his/her eyes. Occlude one nostril at a time, ask the child to say 'yes' if he/she smells anything new, and bring the test smell in from the periphery. Mint or vinegar provide strong smells and are not unpleasant for a child.

II: OPTIC NERVE

An understanding of the basic anatomy of the visual pathways is necessary to interpret your findings (Fig. 7.1). You may be asked to examine any of four aspects of optic nerve integrity:

● visual acuity
● pupils
● visual fields
● fundoscopy.

Visual acuity
This will be dealt with in more depth in Chapter 8, but before examining the cranial nerves it is essential to know if the child is able to see and to have an understanding of the child's ability to comprehend and carry out simple instructions.

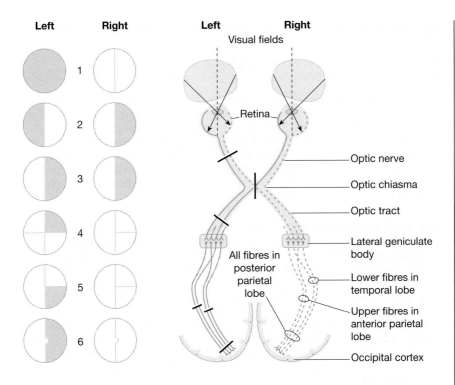

1. Lesion of left optic nerve, leads to complete loss of vision in left eye.

2. Bitemporal hemianopia due to optic chiasma compression.

3. Right homonymous hemianopia from lesion of left optic tract.

4. Upper right quadrantic hemianopia from lesion of lower fibres of optic radiation in the left temporal lobe.

5. Lower quadrantic hemianopia (rare) from lesion of upper fibres of optic radiation in anterior left parietal lobe.

6. Right homonymous hemianopia with macula sparing from a lesion of the optic radiation in the posterior part of the left parietal lobe

Fig. 7.1   Visual field defects.

Pupils

Pupillary responses require intact optic and oculomotor nerves but it is easier to test them at this stage. The pupils should be round, regular and equal on both sides.

Pupillary reflexes   A light is shone on one retina and both pupils should constrict.

- Direct light reflex – pupillary constriction on the stimulated side
- Consensual light reflex – constriction of the pupil on the unstimulated side.

Each eye is tested in turn while the other eye is shielded. The light should be approached from the side to avoid an accommodation response. Occasionally, following initial constriction, the pupil may rapidly alternate between dilatation and constriction. This natural variation is known as 'hippus'.

Accommodation reaction   When the child looks at a near object the eyes converge and the pupils constrict. Accommodation is best tested by asking the child to look at the ceiling and then to focus on your finger held close to their nose.

Abnormal pupillary reflexes   Abnormal responses may occur when there is interruption of the afferent or efferent components of the reflex arc.

Amblyopic light reaction   Afferent defect due to damage of the optic nerve: there is no direct light reflex but a consensual light reflex, as the motor pathway is intact.

Argyll–Robertson pupils – loss of direct and consensual light reflexes but near convergence reflex preserved (midbrain lesion – usually syphilis).

Tonic pupillary reaction   Holmes–Adie pupil – the reaction to light appears absent and there is a a delayed and sustained accommodation reaction. This is a benign condition due to a lesion in the ciliary ganglion, generally encountered in young adult women, and is associated with absent ankle jerks.

Constricted pupils

- Horner's syndrome – this is a sympathetic defect, comprising:
  — partial ptosis
  — pupillary constriction
  — enophthalmos
  — anhidrosis.
  The lesion can occur at different sites: centrally, brain stem or peripherally. The commonest cause in children is iatrogenic, following cardiac surgery.
- Drugs – opiates, cholinesterase inhibitors, rare in the exam!

Dilated pupils (see p. 131 for IIIrd nerve palsy)

- Drugs – sympathomimetics may be used in the exam if fundoscopy is required.
- Blindness – due to damage of the optic nerve.

Unreactive pupils (see p. 131 for IIIrd nerve palsy)

- Cataracts, corneal opacities, vitreous/retinal haemorrhages
- *Do not forget* the prosthetic eye.

Visual fields

Confrontation perimetry   This is the technique required to test the outer limits of the visual fields and is universally badly done.

For older children, sit opposite them, your eyes at the same level as theirs, and explain what you would like them to do. Bring an object from beyond their field of vision and ask them to say 'yes' when they see the object. The important point is that they fix on your eyes, and their responses whilst looking round must be ignored.

Test each eye separately, with one eye closed/covered, then test both eyes together, to exclude sensory inattention.

Test for scotomata   Testing for defects in the central field (scotomata) or an enlarged blind spot is often forgotten but these can be assessed by

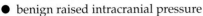

confrontation. With one eye closed, compare your visual field with that of the child, using a small red pin held midway between yourself and the child and asking him/her to focus on your eye. Scotomata are seen in:

- benign raised intracranial pressure
- raised intracranial pressure
- migraine.

For the younger child Confrontation perimetry is possible in an older child of school age but an alternative approach is required for the younger child. Shine a light or show a toy at the periphery of the visual fields and move it around until the child's attention is caught. Eliciting the blink response from different directions is unreliable, as a current of air may act as a corneal stimulus.

Alternatively, the 'distraction' approach can be adopted, involving two examiners. One examiner faces the child, distracting them, while the other examiner brings a toy into the child's peripheral vision from behind. Examiner 1, in front of the child, observes when the child is first aware of the toy.

Menace reflex In a semiconscious child with a gross homonymous hemianopia, or where vision is questionable in an infant, a reflex blink is produced in response to your hand rapidly passing by the eye towards the ear.

Defects of the visual pathway are shown in Figure 7.1. The most common abnormalities in exams are:

- homonymous hemianopia – following a cerebral haemorrhage or neurosurgical procedure
- bitemporal hemianopia – accompanying a pituitary tumour or craniopharyngioma.

Fundoscopy Ask the examiners if you can dim the room lights and pull the curtains. Ask the child to look at a toy held by the parent and explain that you are going to look in to his/her eye. 'Whenever I come between you and the toy, just look through me as if I were not there.' Most children of school age are able to cooperate with this task, at least for a brief period, and it may help if the parent calls the child's name as this provides a useful aural clue as to where he/she should be looking. Look at the right eye from the child's right side using your own right eye and approach from 20º lateral to the point of fixation, as this should bring the optic disc immediately into view. The need to use a plus (red) lens indicates the child has hypermetropia (long-sightedness), whereas a minus (black) lens indicates myopia (short-sightedness). If you have a refractive error, you should correct this with a lens of the ophthalmoscope. A plus lens (e.g. red 10 or 20) should also be used if the anterior chamber is to be examined or if a cataract is suspected. If there is an abnormality, the pupil is likely to have been dilated. The abnormalities you are most likely to see in the exam are described below.

Optic atrophy Only diagnose this if you are certain (see below for myopia):

- inherited, including Leber's disease
- damage to the nerve by tumour or trauma
- following papilloedema or optic neuritis.

Papilloedema   Only diagnose this if you are certain. 'Blurring of the nasal margins' and 'early papilloedema' are for the faint-hearted:

● raised intracranial pressure, including 'benign intracranial hypertension' – usually idiopathic in pubertal girls but other associations are with otitis media, steroid therapy and abnormal plasma calcium
● papillitis, for which the commonest childhood cause is idiopathic optic neuritis.

Both of these aetiologies are associated with a central scotoma, which may be very difficult to demonstrate, and with impaired visual acuity and even blindness.

Choroidoretinitis
● Toxoplasmosis
● Intrauterine rubella or cytomegalovirus.

Retinitis pigmentosa
● Isolated
● Refsum's disease (deafness, ataxia, peripheral neuropathy)
● Laurence–Moon–Biedl syndrome – polydactyly, obesity, hypogonadism, mental retardation.

Cherry red spot   This is a small red spot at the macula (lateral to the optic disc) surrounded by a pale halo. It occurs in a number of the sphingolipidoses:

● Tay–Sachs disease
● Sandhoff's disease
● generalized gangliosidoses
● Niemann–Pick disease.

Beware the child who wears glasses. Most will be short-sighted and the myopic eye has a deep optic cup and temporal pallor. The myopic or short-sighted child can only see distant objects with concave spectacles; the eyeball is relatively large, and may even appear exophthalmic, and the disc seems large and pale ('pseudo-optic atrophy' of myopia). Hypermetropic discs look smaller and may have ill-defined margins but should not be confused with papilloedema. The long-sighted child has a near point which is too far away and therefore requires convex spectacles for near vision. The eyeball is relatively small and the disc is small and pink ('pseudo-papilloedema' of hypermetropia).

III: OCULOMOTOR NERVE, IV: TROCHLEAR NERVE, VI: ABDUCENS

The IIIrd, IVth and VIth nerves control eye movements. Assessment of their function requires an understanding of the anatomy and physiology of the muscles they supply. Involuntary muscle fibres of the third nerve supply the iris and are responsible for pupillary reflexes, and voluntary fibres supply levator palpebrae superioris of the upper eyelid. Six external ocular muscles supply and move the eyeball (Fig. 7.2).

To test eye movements, ask the child to follow your finger with the eyes, keeping the head still. Does the child see two fingers at any point?

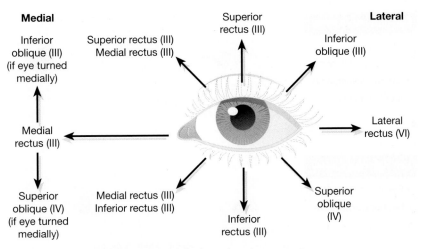

Fig. 7.2 Testing of external ocular movements.

Disorders of ocular movement (Fig. 7.3)
Isolated abnormalities are rare in childhood but paralytic squints make good short cases. Look for scars of previous ophthalmic surgery or neurosurgery. Causes of palsies of these nerves are:

● cerebral palsy
● tumours
● raised intracranial pressure (false localizing sign)
● postmeningitis
● Guillain–Barré syndrome.

Signs of IIIrd nerve palsy (Fig. 7.3a)
● A paralytic divergent squint may be obvious
● The affected eye deviates laterally
● The ipsilateral pupil may be normal or larger and unreactive, depending on the site of the lesion
● Ipsilateral ptosis – ptosis also occurs in Horner's syndrome but the ipsilateral pupil is small. Ptosis may also be congenital (if bilateral, the child tilts the head backwards in order to see), part of a syndrome, traumatic or due to myasthenia gravis
● Demonstrate diplopia, using a pen, except during lateral gaze to the side of the lesion.

Signs of IVth nerve palsy (Fig. 7.3b) The unopposed actions of the
superior oblique muscle are to pull the eye *down* and *out* (best remembered by the mnemonic SODO). The signs of IVth nerve palsy are:

● compensatory torticollis
● a squint is not obvious – test by asking the child to look down while the affected eye is adducted. When the eye is turned medially, downward movements are achieved by the superior oblique (IVth nerve) and elevation by the inferior oblique (IIIrd nerve)
● diplopia occurs on attempted down gaze, causing problems in going down stairs, for example.

Left IIIrd nerve palsy

- Ptosis
- Pupillary dilatation
- Lateral deviation on looking ahead

a

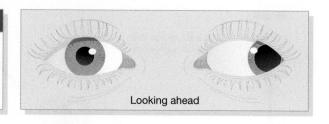

Looking ahead

Left IVth nerve palsy

- Eye turns inwards but not downwards

b

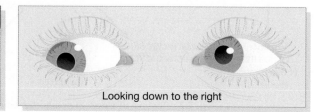

Looking down to the right

Left VIth nerve palsy

- Eye fails to abduct on looking left

c

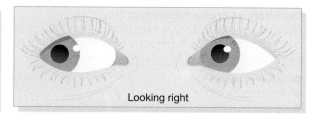

Looking right

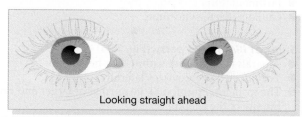

Looking straight ahead

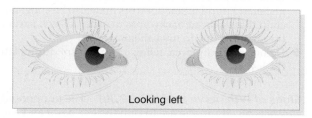

Looking left

Fig. 7.3 Disorders of ocular movements.

Signs of VIth nerve palsy (Fig. 7.3c)

- Convergent squint as the affected eye deviates inwards
- Compensatory torticollis
- Failure of lateral gaze to the affected side.

Internuclear connections

An understanding of the coordination of lateral gaze is important, as internuclear ophthalmoplegia is not insignificantly encountered in the short case exams. A succinct, concise explanation of the problem will impress the examiners.

The medial longitudinal bundle connects the three ocular nerve nuclei to each other and to other nuclei, including the vestibular nuclei, coordinating the activity of the motor nerves to the eye. The parabducens nucleus, in the pons near to the abducens nucleus, coordinates conjugate lateral gaze. Fibres from here run to the VIth nucleus and to the contralateral IIIrd nerve nucleus via the medial longitudinal bundle. Voluntary gaze to the left is initiated in the right frontal cortex (Fig. 7.4).

Internuclear ophthalmoplegia (Fig. 7.4)   This is due to a lesion within the median longitudinal bundle. In a right internuclear opththalmoplegia (INO) there is a lesion of the right median longitudinal bundle. On attempted left lateral gaze, the right eye fails to adduct. The left eye develops coarse nystagmus in abduction. The side of the lesion is on the side of the impaired adduction, not the nystagmus.

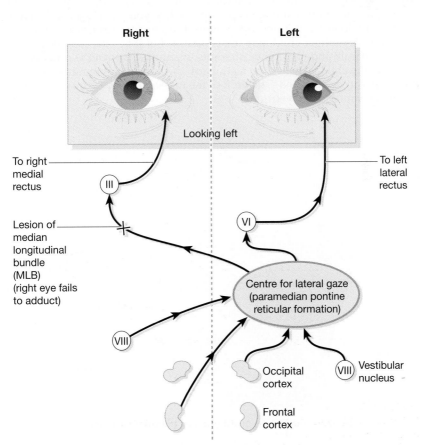

Fig. 7.4   Internuclear ophthalmoplegia.

Destructive frontal lesions, e.g. tumour or infarct, cause failure of conjugate lateral gaze to the side opposite the lesion. In acute lesions, the eyes are often deviated past the midline to the side of the lesion and they therefore look *towards the normal limbs*. There is usually contralateral hemiparesis.

V: TRIGEMINAL NERVE

Sensory component

There are three divisions (with the cutaneous distribution of each division shown in Fig. 7.5):

- ophthalmic
- maxillary
- mandibular.

It is necessary only to test light touch and this can quickly be done by asking children to shut their eyes and to say 'yes' as soon as they feel anything, while you lightly touch (not rub or drag) either side of their face with a wisp of cotton wool, above the eyes, on the cheeks, and either side of the chin.

Motor component

Inspect the muscles of mastication for wasting or fasciculation. Ask the child to open his/her mouth and to keep it open while you push against the chin. In unilateral lower motor neurone lesions, the jaw deviates towards the weak side. A younger child may not cooperate but if he/she can bite on a wooden spatula and resist your attempts to remove it, power is probably intact. As the child clenches the teeth hard, the bulk and symmetry of the masseters can be palpated. The bulk of the masseters may be increased in Duchenne's muscular dystrophy.

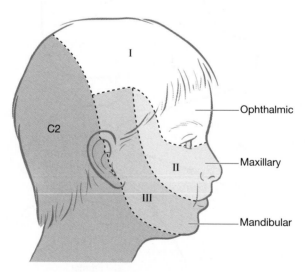

Fig. 7.5 Cutaneous distribution of the trigeminal nerve.

Reflexes

Corneal reflex (sensory V and motor VII)   The sensory afferent limb of this reflex arc is carried in the ophthalmic division of the trigeminal nerve innervating the cornea, while the efferent motor component is supplied by both facial nerves which result in bilateral blinking. This should not be tested in a conscious child as it is unpleasant and unnecessary to assess whether the nerves are intact.

Jaw jerk (motor and sensory V)   This is analogous to the tendon reflexes of the limbs. Both the afferent and efferent pathways are subserved by the trigeminal nerve. The masseter muscle is stretched by placing a thumb on the mandible when the jaw is hanging open; tapping your finger with a tendon hammer will elicit a brisk jaw closure. Increased jaw jerk is only present if there is a bilateral upper motor neurone Vth nerve lesion, e.g. pseudobulbar palsy, which is very rare. Only test for this if other neurological findings are present (Fig. 7.6).

Lesions of the Vth nerve
Trigeminal lesions are very rare in isolation.
   Peripheral
● Trauma
● Tumour of base of the skull
● Herpes zoster infection of the ophthalmic division.
   Central
● Cavernus sinus lesion
● Cerebellopontine tumour
● Bulbar palsy, e.g. motor neurone disease
● Bilateral pseudo bulbar palsy, usually due to hypoxia ischaemia.

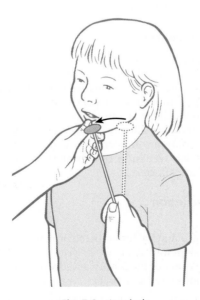

Fig. 7.6   Jaw jerk.

VII: FACIAL NERVE

Motor component
This comprises the muscles of facial expression of the whole of the face. Children should be asked to (it may be necessary to demonstrate these):

- raise their eyebrows
- close their eyes tight shut (remember, the oculomotor and sympathetic nerves supply the muscles which open the eyes; the facial nerve supplies the muscles which close the eyes)
- smile and show you their teeth.

Sensory division
The VIIth supplies taste sensation to the anterior two-thirds of the tongue. This is rarely required to be tested.

Parasympathetic division
This supplies the lacrimal gland. Inability to produce tears is a feature of some of the congenital sensory neuropathies.

Reflexes

Glabella or nasopalpebral reflex   Light percussion with the finger over the root of the nose, or glabella, will elicit a brisk closure of the eyes. In normal people this response will cease after three or four contractions, despite repeated percussion, but it is exaggerated and prolonged in disorders of the extrapyramidal system. Rare in childhood, it is mostly seen in parkinsonism.

Snout reflex   Tapping or stroking of the upper lip, giving rise to puckering or protrusion of the lips, is abnormal beyond infancy and is indicative of a bilateral upper motor neurone lesion.

Lesions of the VIIth nerve (Fig. 7.7)

Upper motor neurone lesion   Above the level of the pons.
   Unilateral lesion   The contralateral side of the face is weak below the level of the eyes but the forehead muscles are normal because they receive bilateral innervation, e.g. tumour or vascular accident.
   Bilateral lesion   May exhibit an obvious snout reflex, lability of emotional expression and occasionally display a strange dissociation between emotion and voluntary movements, e.g. they are able to smile spontaneously, but there is weakness of voluntary facial expression. All muscles on both sides are affected.

Lower motor neurone lesion

   Unilateral lesion
- Asymmetry of the face may be immediately apparent
  — loss of the nasolabial fold
  — drooping of the corner of the mouth and drooling on the affected side.
- No asymmetry obvious – test as above.

All the muscles on the ipsilateral side of the lesion are affected, e.g. Bell's palsy. The lesion can affect any part of the facial nerve, including the facial nerve nucleus in the brain stem.

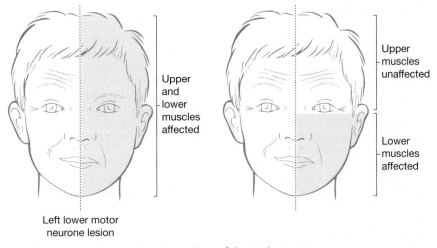

Upper and lower muscles affected

Upper muscles unaffected

Lower muscles affected

Left lower motor neurone lesion

Fig. 7.7 Lesions of the VIIth nerve.

Bilateral lesion This is uncommon:

● Bulbar palsy
● Guillain–Barré syndrome
● Lyme disease.

Bell's palsy An isolated facial nerve palsy of unknown cause is called a Bell's palsy and is the commonest presentation of a cranial nerve lesion in childhood. A lower motor neurone paralysis develops over a few hours, the eye on the affected side cannot be closed and the mouth may be drawn to the opposite side (giving the impression of spasm on the normal side). There may be a sensation of numbness but sensory testing is always normal. Over 90% of children make a complete recovery but this may take up to 3 months. Offer to examine the ears as, rarely, a facial nerve palsy is due to herpes zoster affecting the geniculate ganglion and bullae may be present on the tympanic membrane.

Melkersson syndrome Is a recurrent unilateral or bilateral facial nerve palsy associated with chronic facial oedema. The *Moebius sequence* describes the association of mask-like facies with VIth and VIIth nerve palsies, usually bilateral. Occasionally other cranial nerves are involved and there may also be talipes equinovarus or micrognathia. The Moebius sequence is usually sporadic and is the non-specific end result of a number of different aetiologies, including developmental abnormalities of the brain, peripheral nerve or a myopathy.

Finally, blood pressure should always be checked in a child with a facial nerve palsy, as this may be the first presentation of systemic arterial hypertension.

VIII: VESTIBULOCOCHLEAR (AUDITORY) NERVE

The VIIIth cranial nerve comprises two components: auditory fibres arising from the cochlea, and vestibular fibres arising from the otolith organs and semi-circular canals. It runs alongside the facial nerve in the internal auditory meatus and both enter the brain stem at the cerebellopontine angle. Both may therefore be affected by a posterior fossa tumour or an acoustic neuroma.

Cochlear division

This conveys auditory impulses from the inner ear. Before testing hearing, always examine both external auditory meati for local disease, wax, grommets and damage to the eardrum. Is the child's speech normal? For a description of how to test hearing at different ages, see Chapter 8. If you decide that hearing is impaired, you must try to distinguish whether there is sensorineural (perceptive) deafness, due to damage to the nerve itself, or conductive deafness, due to a lesion within the external auditory meatus or the middle ear. Air conduction is normally more efficient than bone conduction, but when there is a conduction defect, the reverse is true. A tuning fork is used to differentiate the two.

Rinne's test   Place the tuning fork by the child's ear and then place the base of the ringing tuning fork on the mastoid process behind the ear. Ask the child which sounds louder; Rinne is positive if air sound is louder (Fig. 7.8).

● Conductive deafness – bone louder
● Perceptive deafness or normal hearing – air louder.

Weber's lateralizing test   Place a 512-Hz tuning fork on the centre of the child's skull and ask whether it is louder in one ear than the other. Most children of school age can perform this test reproducibly (Fig. 7.8).

● Conductive deafness – louder on the diseased side
● Perceptive deafness – louder on the healthy side.

A guide to interpreting the results of the tuning fork tests is given in Table 7.2 and differences between sensorineural and conductive deafness are highlighted in Table 7.3. The severity of the hearing loss is as follows:

● mild loss: 20–30 dB
● moderate: 30–50 dB
● severe: 50–70 dB
● profound: 70–90 dB.

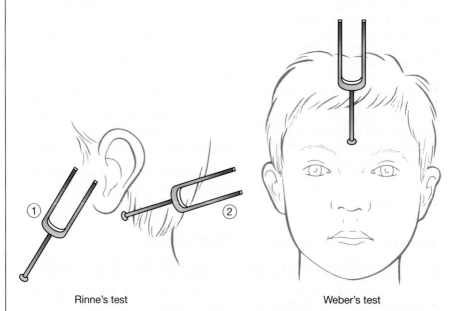

Rinne's test   Weber's test

Fig. 7.8   Hearing tests.

Table 7.2 To determine whether the hearing loss is sensorineural or conductive

Right		Left	Interpretation
Rinne positive	Weber central	Rinne positive	Normal or severe bilateral sensorineural loss
Rinne positive	Weber left	Rinne negative	Left conductive or mixed hearing loss
Rinne negative	Weber central	Rinne negative	Bilateral mixed or conductive deafness
Rinne positive	Weber right	Rinne negative	Left severe or profound sensorineural loss

Table 7.3 Differences between sensorineural and conductive deafness

Sensorineural deafness	Conductive deafness
Cochlear, nerve, brain stem or auditory cortex disease	Foreign body or middle ear disease
Rare	Common
Often severe	Usually mild
High tones lost first (>60 dB)	Low tones lost first (<60 dB)
Loss of consonants (high frequencies)	Loss of vowels (low frequencies)
Often congenital and permanent	Usually acquired and transient
May be a family history of deafness	
Mumps is commonest cause in >5 years	

Causes of deafness

Conductive deafness
● Chronic secretory otitis media (glue ear).

Perceptive deafness   *Prenatal* causes (60%) include:
● inherited (50%) – may be isolated or part of a syndrome, e.g. Pendred's syndrome (autosomal recessive), Waardenburg's syndrome (autosomal dominant), oto-palato-digital syndrome (X-linked)
● intrauterine infection – *Toxoplasma*, rubella, cytomegalovirus, syphilis
● congenital malformations of the ear.

Perinatal causes (10%) include:
● birth asphyxia
● kernicterus
● aminoglycosides.

Postnatal causes (30%) include:
● meningitis
● encephalitis
● trauma
● ototoxic drugs.

Therefore, consider deafness in any of the following groups of children (see Ch. 8):

● family history of deafness
● low birthweight

- cleft palate
- cerebral palsy
- global developmental delay
- delayed language milestones
- history of recurrent ear infections or central nervous system infection
- the parents are concerned that the child is deaf.

Vestibular division

This conveys postural sensation from the labyrinth of the inner ear. It is therefore tested along with cerebellar function in the assessment of balance and gait (see previous section). Damage to the vestibular nerve or nucleus may also produce nystagmus.

Nystagmus Nystagmus is characterized by involuntary oscillations of the eye, which may be horizontal, vertical or rotatory. Nystagmus should be observed for when testing ocular movements. It is defined by the direction of the fast phase, but it is the slow phase which is pathological. Ask the child to fix on your finger (more than 2 feet away, to avoid the interference of convergence) and move your finger through a clock face from 3 to 9, then from 6 to 12 o'clock for 5 seconds at each position. If nystagmus is present, the eye will drift away from fixation and it must be sustained for more than a few beats. A few beats of nystagmus at extremes of gaze are normal. Nystagmus is caused by a lesion of the cerebellum, brain stem, cervical cord or inner ear. Always offer to examine hearing, cerebellar function and the ocular fundi.

Central nystagmus
- Results from brain stem lesions, e.g. vertebrobasilar ischaemia, phenytoin toxicity
- Nystagmus in *any* direction:
  — up-beat nystagmus: lesion in floor of fourth ventricle, pontine tegmentum
  — down-beat nystagmus: extrinsic compressive lesion of foramen magnum.

Cerebellar nystagmus Nystagmus is *towards* the side of the lesion

Vestibular nystagmus
- Only in *one* direction of gaze
- Nystagmus is *away* from the side of the lesion
- Made worse by gaze in that direction (Alexander's law)
- Horizontal or rotational but not vertical
- May be associated with tinnitus and deafness.

Positional nystagmus
- Occurs in benign positional vertigo (BPV) and is brought on by rapid head movements often associated with a delay of a few seconds and fatiguability (Hallpike's test)
- May follow head injury or viral labyrinthitis
- Occurs in only one direction.

Ocular nystagmus
- Due to poor macular vision which impairs retinal fixation
- Often rotatory on central fixation but can be pendular
- Frequently congenital.

Ataxic nystagmus Occurs in internuclear ophthalmoplegia due to a gaze palsy. The adducting eye does not move and there is nystagmus of the abducting eye.

See-saw nystagmus
- One eye rises and turns in; other eye falls and turns out
- Occurs in parasellar tumours.

Optokinetic nystagmus Can be induced in normal children (Catford drum or a car passing fence poles).

Congenital nystagmus Rapid rhythmic eye movements with normal vision. The cause is unknown and is sometimes familial. The rest of the examination is normal and the condition may improve with age.

IX: GLOSSOPHARYNGEAL NERVE

Motor division
The IXth nerve supplies the stylopharyngeus muscle, which elevates the upper pharynx, together with the palatopharyngeal muscle, which is supplied by the Xth nerve. This is difficult to test because the child will still be able to elevate the palate if the Xth nerve is intact.

Sensory division
The majority of the IXth nerve functions are combined with the Xth nerve, except for taste, which can be tested in isolation but is rarely done in exams. The IXth nerve supplies sensation from the nasopharynx and soft palate and taste from the posterior third of the tongue.

X: VAGUS NERVE

The IXth and Xth nerves are usually considered together as they exit the skull together, run a similar course, and both are usually involved in a single lesion.

Motor division
Motor fibres supply the voluntary muscles of the pharynx and larynx. The parasympathetic fibres supply the heart, lungs and abdominal viscera.

Reflexes

Gag reflex The afferent arm is supplied by the glossopharyngeal nerve and the efferent arm, the vagus nerve. This test should not be elicited in a conscious child.

Palatal reflex Innervation is as for gag reflex. The soft palate elevates when touched. When testing these reflexes, the stimulus should be applied to each side in turn (Fig. 7.9). Dysarthria, nasal speech and difficulty in swallowing are clues to dysfunction of these nerves.

Apart from damage to the recurrent laryngeal branch of the vagus nerve, isolated lesions of the IXth and Xth nerves are rare, but both may be damaged in posterior fossa tumours, basal meningitis, syringobulbia and fractures to the base of the skull. Unilateral lesions cause the palatal arch on the affected side to droop, and it does not elevate when the child says 'ah'. Asymmetry of the movements of the palatal arches may persist for months after tonsillectomy, but speech and swallowing are unaffected.

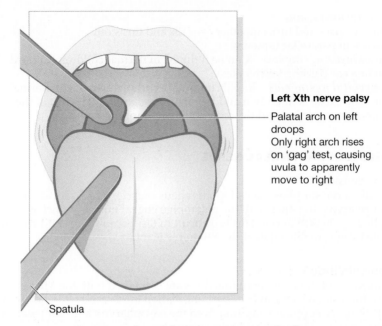

Left Xth nerve palsy

Palatal arch on left
droops
Only right arch rises
on 'gag' test, causing
uvula to apparently
move to right

Spatula

Fig. 7.9   Lesion of the Xth nerve – palatal reflex.

XI: SPINAL ACCESSORY NERVE

This innervates the trapezius and sternocleidomastoid muscles. Function is easily tested by asking children to:

● shrug their shoulders (Fig. 7.10).
● turn their head to one side, while you place your hand on the medial side of the jaw, and ask them to push against you. This tests the sternocleidomastoid on the opposite side to which the head is turned.

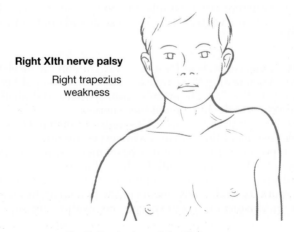

Right XIth nerve palsy

Right trapezius
weakness

Fig. 7.10   Lesion of the XIth nerve.

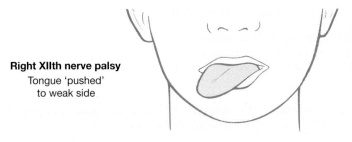

Right XIIth nerve palsy
Tongue 'pushed'
to weak side

Fig. 7.11 Lesion of the XIIth nerve.

Younger children may not cooperate but will obligingly turn towards a toy or their mother's voice.

XII: HYPOGLOSSAL NERVE

This supplies the muscles of the tongue. First inspect the tongue lying at rest in the floor of the mouth for spontaneous fasciculation, a sign of lower motor neurone disease, sometimes apparent in children with one of the spinal muscular atrophies. (A word of warning: perfectly healthy children find it impossible to hold their tongue absolutely still so make sure you look at a few 'normals'.) Now ask the child to stick out his/her tongue. A unilateral lesion causes ipsilateral atropy and deviation of the tongue to the affected side. Do not mistake an apparent deviation of the tongue, due to the mouth being twisted as in a facial nerve palsy, for a real deviation (Fig. 7.11).

Upper motor neurone lesions of the hypoglossal nerve (small spastic tongue) are extremely rare in childhood, except in cerebral palsy.

NEUROLOGICAL EXAMINATION OF A BABY/TODDLER

The emphasis is partly determined by the conditions likely to be encountered in the DCH or MRCPCH examinations in this age group:

- dysmorphic children
- hydrocephalus
- other abnormalities of the head
- cerebral palsy
- neural tube defects
- hypotonia.

Apart from abnormalities affecting the eyes, you are very unlikely to see cranial nerve problems in this age group and you are unlikely to be asked to test sensation.

INSPECTION

A great deal of information will be gleaned from observing the infant carefully. Rushing straight in to undress the child and test the tone and power in the arms will upset the child and prevent further assessment. Start with the child fully dressed on a parent's lap.

143

Overall size and proportions of head/trunk/limbs

Obvious dysmorphic features (see Ch. 11)

Carefully examine for any features suggestive of a neurocutaneous syndrome (see pp. 212, 242–245). You may need to wait until the child is undressed.

Ataxic telangiectasia Conjunctival telangiectasia usually appears by 5 years and later becomes apparent on the cheeks.

Tuberous sclerosis Adenoma sebaceum is not present in the very young child but appears after 4–5 years of age.

Neurofibromatosis type I (von Recklinghausen's disease) In postpubertal individuals with proven neurofibromatosis type I, 75% have six or more café-au-lait spots of more than 1.5 cm diameter. Among normal people, 10% have one to five café-au-lait spots of more than 1.5 cm size. In normal children under 5 years old, only 0.75% have more than two café-au-lait macules larger than 1.5 cm.

Sturge–Weber syndrome A port-wine stain affecting the area of one or more divisions of the trigeminal nerve, usually the ophthalmic division, is present from birth; 30% have a contralateral hemiplegia and 30% have learning difficulties, although learning difficulties are only present if the child has epilepsy.

Posture

A consistently maintained asymmetric posture should always arouse suspicion. The typical posture in the newborn is one of flexion. Look for the following:

Torticollis Abnormal posture of the head may be accompanied by a squint or hemianopia. Torticollis is most common in a young infant due to sternocleidomastoid tumour but may also be due to hemivertebrae, cervical adenitis and ocular muscle imbalance.

    Sternocleidomastoid 'tumour' An ischaemic contracture of the muscle, sometimes due to a birth injury, causes ipsilateral lateral neck flexion and rotation of the chin to the opposite side.

    A paralytic squint The new position of the head allows both eyes to fixate.

Spinal curvature (scoliosis, kyphosis, lordosis) Lumbar lordosis may be particularly obvious, and quite normal, in thin girls.

Hypotonia The child may sit on the lower end of the back instead of on the buttocks, while a floppy baby may show the 'frog legs' posture when lying supine. Regional hypotonia may also occur, e.g. in Erb's palsy (p. 151) or spina bifida (p. 153, 178).

Hypertonia Asymmetrical posture of the freely hanging legs may be the first sign of unilateral weakness or spasticity.

Generalized hypertonia The legs are usually more affected than the arms, the trunk tends to be opisthotonic, and the extensor tone in the neck results in seemingly good head control in ventral suspension but poor head control on pulling to sit. The legs are in extension with the arms flexed.

Opisthotonus This must not be confused with neck stiffness, which you are unlikely to see in an exam situation. Opisthotonus is an involuntary extension of the neck accompanied by arching of the back due to spasm of the erector spinae.
Causes are:

- cerebral palsy
- acute and severe meningeal or cerebral irritation
- tetanus.

Neck stiffness is an unwillingness to flex the neck as this stretches the meninges causing pain if they are inflamed. It is an unreliable sign in infants and toddlers and is best assessed by placing a parent or toy at the outside of the child's visual field and asking the child to look for it. The more conventional approach is to palpate the back of the neck with the fingertips while flexing the neck. However, many normal children will resist this manoeuvre.

Movement
Observe the quantity and quality of both gross movements involving trunk and limbs and fine movements of the face, fingers and feet. Can the child sit or stand?
Movement can be divided into the following:
General paucity
Asymmetrical
Accessory
- Tic – an identical movement repeated, i.e. a habit
- Tremor – involuntary, rhythmical alternating movement. May occur at rest or only on reaching for an object (intention tremor of cerebellar disease)
- Titubation – tremor of the head and neck
- Chorea – rapid, involuntary, irregular movements, usually of the extremities or face, which may interfere with speech or gait. The movements increase with effort or excitement. The causes in childhood, which are all rare, are:
  — anticonvulsant side-effect
  — benign hereditary chorea
  — Wilson's disease
  — juvenile-onset Huntington's chorea
  — Sydenham's chorea
- Athetoid – slow, involuntary, writhing movements, usually of the proximal limbs. The commonest cause is cerebral palsy, but basal ganglia disease, in particular Wilson's disease, must be excluded
- Convulsive – movements generalized, localized or flexion spasms ('Salaam attacks') of myoclonic epilepsy.

Having spent a few moments observing the overall appearance of the child, it is simply a matter of starting at the top and working downwards.

EYES

Always start with examination of the eyes because, should the baby begin to cry, observation of the eyes becomes impossible (see Ch. 8 for further description of examination of the eyes). Eye-to-eye contact establishes rapport and it is said that children can spot a friendly candidate by the expression in the candidate's eyes!

Fixation Does he fixate?

Nystagmus (see pp. 140–141) Is there spontaneous nystagmus?

Ptosis *Unilateral* ptosis may be due to a Horner's syndrome (pupil small) or IIIrd nerve lesion (pupil large and paralytic squint). The most likely cause in this age group is a congenital Horner's syndrome as a result of shoulder traction at birth damaging the sympathetic chain.

Bilateral ptosis is more likely to be due to a myopathy than to myasthenia in this age group. Look for other evidence of myopathy:

- restricted eye movements
- long, thin face
- drooping mouth
- lack of expression
- thin
- may be breathless
- kyphosis/scoliosis.

Possible causes are:

- nemaline rod myopathy
- centronuclear myopathy
- congenital myotonic dystrophy.

Eyeballs Are the eyeballs apparently equal in size? The eyeball may be prominent (exophthalmos, e.g. thyrotoxicosis), sunken (enophthalmos, e.g. Horner's syndrome) or enlarged (congenital or acquired buphthalmos).

Is there conjunctivitis, icterus, haemorrhage, abnormal iris pigmentation, Brushfield spots, colobomata or aniridia?

Pupils Are the pupils equal in size? A large pupil may be associated with amblyopia or a lesion of the oculomotor nerve (see p. 131); a small pupil with Horner's syndrome.

External ocular movements Test the range of eye movements in the four cardinal directions by moving an interesting toy around in the child's field of view. Are the eye movements conjugate? Does the child have a squint (see p. 197)? Most children can follow an object through 180° by 4 months.

Fundoscopy and assessment of pupillary reflexes, visual fields and visual acuity These should all be left until the end of the examination unless you have noted some abnormality.

Other cranial nerves
Look for a facial nerve palsy. In this age group, this will almost certainly be a lower motor neurone lesion (therefore affecting the whole of one-half of the face) related to birth trauma. The corner of the mouth on the intact side is pulled up during smiling or crying.

Other cranial nerve lesions are rare and difficult to test but there are a few simple clues.

- The ability to suck and swallow in a coordinated and effective way is present from about 35 weeks' gestation and implies normal function of nerves VII, IX, X and XII.
- Listen to the child's speech:
  — *Delayed*: speech may be delayed in mental retardation (see p. 192) or autism, may lack intelligibility in cerebral palsy, or be a stammering, monotone in deafness. Normal articulation makes lesions of VII, X and XII unlikely
  — *Dysarthria*: beware of diagnosing dysarthria as there are wide variations of normality in pre-school children.
  — *Dysphonia/aphonia*: dysphonia, a whispering, high-pitched voice or cry, or aphonia suggests damage to the recurrent laryngeal branch of the Xth cranial nerve. Aphonia may also occur because of chorea affecting the tongue or facial muscles. In the pre-verbal child, listen for the high-pitched cry of cerebral irritation or injury, the peculiar meowing cry of cri-du-chat syndrome, the hoarse cry of congenital hypothyroidism, and the crowing cry associated with laryngeal narrowing. The 'good' baby who 'never cries' may be profoundly delayed.
- Symmetrical appearance and movement of the tongue requires an intact XIIth nerve.

If other signs deem it appropriate, you may offer to test the corneal reflex (sensory limb is V, motor limb is VII) or the gag reflex (sensory limb is IX, motor limb is X) but neither of these unpleasant tests should be performed routinely. Lesions of IX and X usually occur together and suggest a bulbar palsy due to a posterior fossa abnormality or a pseudobulbar palsy (upper motor neurone lesion), most frequently associated with cerebral palsy.

HEAD

Shapes (Fig. 7.12)

Plagiocephaly From above, the head appears as a parallelogram.

- Most often a 'postural' deformity which corrects spontaneously once the child is mobile
- Unilateral coronal synostosis.

Scaphocephaly The head is long in the anteroposterior diameter and narrow when viewed from the front (also called dolichocephaly).

- Usually associated with prematurity
- Sagittal synostosis
- Sometimes Hurler's syndrome.

Turricephaly The head is tall due to compensatory upward growth (also called acrocephaly). Raised intracranial pressure is especially likely to occur with this deformity.

- Bilateral coronal synostosis – think of Apert's syndrome and Carpenter's syndrome.

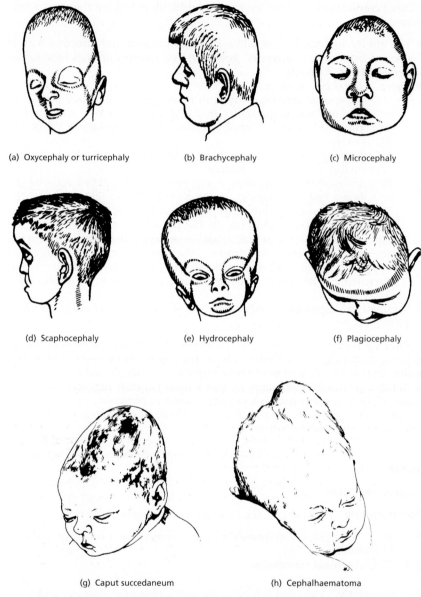

(a) Oxycephaly or turricephaly   (b) Brachycephaly   (c) Microcephaly

(d) Scaphocephaly   (e) Hydrocephaly   (f) Plagiocephaly

(g) Caput succedaneum   (h) Cephalhaematoma

Fig. 7.12 Head shapes. (Reproduced with permission from Forfar J O, Arneil G C (eds) 1984 Textbook of paediatrics, 3rd edn. Churchill Livingstone, Edinburgh.)

Brachycephaly   The back of the head is flattened.

● Down's syndrome
● Bilateral coronal synostosis.

Sutures
● Coronal
● Sagittal

- Lambdoid
- Metopic – in the midline of the forehead due to early synostosis between the frontal bones; cosmetic problem only.

If premature fusion of a suture occurs, skull growth cannot occur perpendicular to that suture but continues to occur in the line of the fused suture; hence sagittal fusion results in scaphocephaly. Widely separated sutures suggest raised intracranial pressure (see below), as do distended scalp veins (unless there is superior vena caval obstruction).

Fontanelles
- Anterior – diamond shape
- Posterior – triangular
- Third fontanelle – may be only a barely perceptible widening of the sagittal suture between anterior and posterior fontanelles. This is a normal variant but also a clue to Down's syndrome in the newborn.

Fontanelles usually close at around 1 year of age. Delayed closure (more than 18 months) suggests:

- hydrocephalus
- Down's syndrome
- hypothyroidism.

Abnormally wide fontanelles at any age suggest:

- rickets
- hypothyroidism
- cranial synostosis
- rare syndromes such as Smith–Lemli–Opitz syndrome, Zellweger's syndrome and Rubinstein–Taybi syndrome.

The mean anterior fontanelle measurement (length plus width divided by 2) is 2 cm at birth, but the 95% confidence limits during the first year of life are 0–5 cm. In contrast to this wide range, the posterior fontanelle is fingertip size or smaller in 97% of newborn infants.

Intracranial pressure is best assessed by appearance and palpation of the anterior fontanelle, provided the infant is sitting up and not crying. The fontanelle may be:

- bulging – elevated above the convexity of the skull
- tense – flush with the skull but there is increased resistance to light pressure with the fingertips and pulsation at cardiac frequency is easily felt
- normal
- sunken – implies 5–10% dehydration.

Head size

Occipitofrontal circumference (OFC)   Leave OFC measurement until the end.

Microcephaly and macrocephaly   These are discussed in the short cases at the end of the chapter (pp. 176–178).

Ventriculoperitoneal shunt/reservoir
Look carefully for the presence of a shunt or reservoir, especially if the child has a large head.

HANDS

Dysmorphism
- Syndactyly
- Polydactyly
- Clinodactyly
- Abnormal palmar creases.

Muscle wasting
This can be difficult in chubby hands of babies and toddlers.

Handedness
- Usually becomes obvious between the ages of $1\frac{1}{2}$–5 years.
- Hand preference in a young child under 18 months of age requires a careful search for other evidence of hemiplegia.

Textbooks often make the observation that much can be learned from watching a child play with a toy or scribbling, without actually telling you what exactly can be learned. Such observations tell you about:

- symmetry
- skills which have to be learned and are age-dependent
- coordination (e.g. threading beads), which again is age-dependent.

Unfortunately, it may take a long time to get a young child to cooperate by playing or drawing for a stranger, time which is certainly not available in the short cases. The best compromise is to proffer an interesting toy and observe:

- Does the child reach out for it?
- Is there an intention tremor?
- What sort of grasp does the child have?
- Does the child transfer between hands or indulge in mouthing?
- Is there symmetry of range of movement between both hands and arms?

NOW UNDRESS TO THE NAPPY

A child still in nappies beyond the age of 3 years is unusual and this is worthy of comment and may be a clue to an organic problem of sphincter control. Undressing provides much information about a baby's tone and about an older child's dexterity. Although most 3-year-olds should be able to undress with a little help, they may be reluctant to do so in the presence of a stranger and may not want your help. While undressing the child, also look for:

- muscle wasting – generalized or specific
- scars
- ventriculoperitoneal or ventriculo-atrial shunts
- scoliosis
- lower spine abnormalities.

ARMS

Inspection
Look for the following.

Deformity Bony or soft tissue?

Muscle bulk
- Difficult to assess as toddlers have plenty of subcutaneous fat
- Loss of bulk may be due to a lower motor neurone lesion, disuse atrophy or generalized wasting.

Posture
- Shoulder adducted, elbow flexed, wrist flexed and hand clenched suggest a pyramidal tract problem (usually cerebral palsy).
- Shoulder adducted and internally rotated, elbow extended and wrist flexed (waiter's tip posture) are characteristic of upper brachial plexus lesion (Erb's palsy, usually a sequel to shoulder dystocia at birth).
- A 'claw hand' is consistent with either a lower brachial plexus or radial nerve injury, or arthrogryphosis, in which case other joints will be involved.

Only when you have obtained as much information as possible from inspection should you proceed to the remainder of the examination of the upper limbs.

Tone
Tone is defined as resistance to passive movement. Always compare both sides, looking for any signs of asymmetry.

Handling the child will give a general idea of muscle tone. A useful technique is lightly to hold both of the child's wrists in your hands and quickly shake them to and fro, watching how freely the hands 'waggle'. Again, a difference between the two sides is the clue here.

Hypertonia   Increased tone is indicated by excessive firmness of the muscles and stiffness in movements of the limbs. There are two distinct types, *spasticity* and *rigidity*. In children, it is almost always spasticity rather than rigidity and reflects an upper motor neurone lesion, most frequently cerebral palsy. It is characterized by a rapid build-up in resistance during the first few degrees of passive movement and then, as the movement continues, there is a sudden lessening of resistance, referred to as 'clasp-knife' spasticity. Rigidity is the term used to describe sustained resistance to passive movement, occurring in diseases of the basal ganglia, and is similar to the sensation produced by bending a lead pipe. This phenomenon is referred to as 'lead pipe' or extrapyramidal rigidity.

Hypotonia   This is indicated by softness of the muscles, floppiness on handling or laxity of the joints. Hypotonia may be due to a lower motor neurone lesion (spinal cord or more rarely peripheral nerve), a problem with the neuromuscular junction or the muscle, or simply due to muscle wasting in a child with severe failure to thrive. Confusingly, 'central' hypotonia may also occur in children with a higher disorder of tone control (see short cases), including atonic cerebral palsy.

Clonus   This describes a rhythmic series of involuntary muscle contractions evoked by stretching the muscle.

- A few beats are seen in normal, anxious patients
- Sustained clonus
  — more than three beats is significant
  — continues throughout muscle stretching, but is aborted by further stretching – that is how to differentiate between spontaneous sustained clonus and seizure

— 'hard' neurological sign
— reflects exaggerated tendon reflexes as a result of damage to the upper motor neurones
● Most commonly evoked at the ankle or knee joint.

Power
● Impossible to test formally in this age group
● Hand preference may be due to a problem of tone, power or coordination and these are difficult to dissociate
● A clue to power in the hand muscles is provided by:
— tightness with which the child will grip an object
— a trick for assessing flexor power in the arms is to pull the infant up by the arms from a supine position; an infant with normal power will flex at the elbows to resist your pull.

Coordination
This is best assessed by observing play as discussed above. Remember that coordination will also be impaired by poor visual acuity, cerebellar problems (ataxic cerebral palsy or posterior fossa tumour) or sensory loss (very rare).

Reflexes
The testing of reflexes should be omitted until the end of your examination, as striking children with a tendon hammer is not guaranteed to endear you to them. See examination of the reflexes (p. 156).

Sensation
This is impossible to test in a young child except by demonstration of withdrawal from a painful stimulus, a technique which should never be used in exams. Good coordination requires normal sensation in the hands and fingers.

TRUNK

Muscle weakness
A pot belly and lumbar lordosis are normal in toddlers, but if either is extreme this may be due to muscle weakness.

Proximal weakness
All children over 18 months should be able to get to their feet from the supine position, and difficulty in doing so may be a sign of proximal weakness (Gower's sign). Children over 6 years should be able to sit up from the supine position with hands folded across the abdomen.

Truncal ataxia
All children over 10 months should be able to sit unsupported and failure to do so may be due to weakness or truncal ataxia.

Balance
With the child sitting and his/her head central, give a gentle sideways push against the shoulder. Normal children will keep their balance by shifting their weight to the side of the push. If the child falls sideways and has to be

caught, or is dependent on the hands for lateral support, there may be an abnormality of tone or posture.

Cerebellar ataxia
This is particularly suggested by swaying movements. With the child in the same position, catch his/her interest with a small toy and move it through 180º. If children aged over 3 years cannot turn to the toy except by supporting themselves on their hands or altering their seating position, truncal balance or muscle tone may be deficient.

Skin examination
Again examine the skin for evidence of phakomatoses (see also Ch. 9 and p. 242).

Tuberous sclerosis   Ash-leaf depigmentation and darker brown café-au-lait patches may occur anywhere on the trunk and a shagreen patch, a thickened area of skin, may be present over the lumbosacral area. Small fibromata particularly occur under the toenails. Adenoma sebaceum lesions appear on the face after 4–5 years of age.

Neurofibromatosis type I   Café-au-lait patches may appear in early infancy before the manifestation of cutaneous neurofibromata and neurological signs. More than six café-au-lait spots, each more than 1.5 cm in diameter, are considered significant. Axillary freckling is also a feature of this condition.

BACK

Turn the child over and expose the sacrum and buttocks. Look for muscle wasting and examine for:

● obvious neural tube defect – is it a meningocele or meningomyelocele? Rarely, a meningocele may be completely covered by skin. Define the extent of the lesion
● if there is no obvious abnormality of the spine, quickly run your finger along the spinous processes to detect spina bifida occulta
● dural sinus – usually sacral but may be thoracic or cervical. Sacral dimples are common and a true sinus is rare. Clues to distinguishing these are:
— if you can see the base of the defect, it is not a sinus
— if it is low on the sacrum, in the midline, and not associated with a naevus or hairy patch, it is unlikely to be a sinus
● a tuft of hair, dimple or naevus may also overlie a diastometamyelia
● Mongolian blue spots are common over the buttocks and sacrum of all dark-skinned children

It is important to examine the back before the legs as the former may give a clue to the latter.

LEGS

Follow the same sequence as for the upper limbs, starting with inspection. This is most easily accomplished by getting a toddler to walk towards a parent.

Gait

Toe walking   A normal variant in the development of some children is to walk for a time on their tip-toes. However, check that there are no contractures by demonstrating the normal range of passive dorsiflexion at the ankle. Toe walking may also be the first clue to subtle *spastic diplegia*.

In-toe (pigeon toes) and out-toe (duck's feet)   These gaits are common, normal variants in toddlers.

Bow legs (genu varum)   Again, this is normal in toddlers, but if bowing is extreme:

● look for signs of rickets at the wrists and ribs
● ask about a family history, and look for blue sclerae and hypermobile joints (osteogenesis imperfecta)
● look for achondroplasia.

Blount's disease (an acquired abnormality of the proximal tibial metaphysis) may cause unilateral bowing.

Knock-knees (genu valgum)   This often develops in pre-school children as their bow legs resolve and is usually accompanied by flat feet (pes planus). If the valgus deformity is severe, again think of rickets and if severe pes planus occurs in isolation, look for evidence of weakness or hypermobility.

Broad-based gait   This is normal in toddlers. Cerebellar ataxia and certain cerebral palsies cause a wide-based gait.

Waddling   Untreated bilateral congenital dislocation of the hip is rare nowadays. Pelvic girdle weakness, as in Duchenne's muscular dystrophy, may also cause a waddling gait, as may the abnormal pelvic tilt in achondroplasia and Morquio–Brailsford syndrome, both of which exhibit short stature.

Hemiplegic gait   There is increased tone in a pyramidal distribution (hip adducted and extended, knee extended, ankle plantarflexed) so that the affected leg is held straight and moved stiffly, and forward motion is achieved by circumduction, the foot scraping the floor, rather than by flexion at the hip and knee. This gives the appearance of walking on the toes of the affected side. There is limited swinging of the arm on the same side with elbow flexion.

Spastic diplegia   Walking is achieved with the hips and knees semiflexed. The gait is stiff-legged and scissoring. Classically, if the child is crawling on the knees, the feet are held off the floor.

Limp   This term describes any gait where less time is spent bearing weight on one leg than on the other (see p. 232).

If the gait is found to be abnormal, examine the legs for deformities, surgical scars, rashes and joint swelling and proceed to assess the range of movements at ankle, knee and hip joints after enquiring about the site of any pain.

Deformity

Bulk
- Generalized bilateral wasting in spina bifida
- Bilateral wasting, particularly proximally, in Werdnig–Hoffmann disease
- Unilateral wasting in hemiplegia
- Hemihypertrophy – measure thigh and calf girth at fixed distances above and below both knees
- Bilateral calf hypertrophy (but also weakness, hence 'pseudohypertrophy') in Duchenne's muscular dystrophy.

Fasciculation
- Rarely seen in infants
- May be seen when there is muscle wasting
- Produced by spontaneous contractions of large groups of muscle fibres or of whole motor units
- Suggests a lower motor neurone lesion lying proximally, near the anterior horn cells, e.g. motor neurone disease
- It is not always present when there is denervation
- Can be seen in normal people but there is no associated muscle wasting and the movements are more coarse, e.g. affecting the thighs after exercise.

Posture
- *'Frog's legs'* – the child lies with hips abducted and knees flexed. This is a sign of hypotonia, rather than weakness, in the legs (see short case, 'The floppy infant', p. 175)
- *Scissoring* – the legs are dystonic and cross over, particularly when the child is held supported under the arms. Scissoring is often seen when there is adductor spasm, as in cerebral diplegia
- *Hemiplegic* – the affected leg may be held extended in severe cases but spastic hemiplegia is often only apparent on examination and not on inspection.

Tone
Clinically, tone is the resistance felt when a joint is moved passively. When a person is normally relaxed, manipulation of a joint evokes a slight, elastic resistance from the adjacent muscles. This degree of normal tension can only be gauged by repeated examination, and abnormalities of tone can be difficult to evaluate. Lightly lift each leg and try to flex it at the knee and hip a few times, assessing the degree of resistance you have to overcome. Alternatively, try 'flicking' the knee joints off the bed; normally, flexion will occur at the knee and the heel will remain in contact with the mattress, but if spasticity is present, the whole leg is jerked into the air and remains straight. Also try to abduct each hip with the knee held flexed. It is important that the pelvis is held fixed with one hand so that movements of the pelvis do not compensate for limitation of movement at the hip. Tone may be increased or decreased (p. 151).

Clonus   Do not forget to check for clonus (pp. 151–152).

Power
Power can be partly gauged from the *gait*.

Independent walking   This is normally achieved between 10 and 18 months.

Delayed walking

Commonest causes
- 'Bottom shuffling' – ask about family history of bottom shuffling
- Familial delay.

Rarer causes
- Weakness – if distal, children may drag their feet when they walk
- Neuromuscular wasting
- Wasting due to failure to thrive
- Deformity
- Mental retardation.

Regression Check for regression of previously normal walking.

Power may also be assessed in an infant by *passively flexing the legs* as for examining tone and observing how hard the infant pushes against you.

Pelvic girdle power The ability to stand up from a lying position requires good power in both legs and in the pelvic girdle muscles. Although Gower's sign is classically a sign of Duchenne's muscular dystrophy, it may be present in any child with marked proximal weakness.

Coordination

A normal gait obviously implies good coordination but progressively more sensitive tests are tackling stairs, running and hopping.

REFLEXES

Tendon reflexes

All the reflexes should be assessed at the end of the neurological examination. Asking a pre-school child to relax looks foolish on your part and is a complete waste of time even in older children. However, talking to the child and asking questions may provide enough distraction for you to sneak in that vital tap from the tendon hammer. There is little to be gained from using a smaller hammer for smaller children so just try to become proficient with the standard hammer. Hold the hammer by the end of the handle but not as though it is a hammer!

- *Biceps and triceps reflexes* are elicited with the arm flexed at the elbow. It is easier to elicit the biceps jerk by placing your own thumb over the radial insertion of the biceps tendon and striking your thumb rather than the tendon directly, which is hard to find in a chubby arm.
- *Supinator jerk* is difficult to obtain in a young child, adds little to the information from testing the biceps, and may be painful.
- *The knee jerks* are most easily compared by supporting both legs with your left arm and tapping below both patellae in quick succession.
- *Ankle jerks* can be elicited either by putting the legs into the 'frog' position and tapping each Achilles tendon in turn, or by placing your fingertips on the ball of the foot and striking your fingers.

Root levels of reflexes These are easily remembered because, in the order of testing, the levels descend from 8 to 1.

- Triceps – C7,8
- Biceps – C5,6

- Supinator – C5,6
- Knee – L3,4
- Ankle – S1,2.

There are seven cervical vertebrae, 12 thoracic vertebrae, five lumbar vertebrae, five sacral vertebrae (fused to form the sacrum) and four coccygeal vertebrae (the lower three are commonly fused). There are 31 pairs of spinal nerves that leave the spinal cord and pass through intervertebral foramina in the vertebral column. The spinal nerves are named according to the regions of the vertebral column with which they are associated: eight cervical (although there are seven vertebrae), 12 thoracic, five lumbar, five sacral and one coccygeal (although there are four coccygeal vertebrae). The spinal cord terminates at the level of the lower border of the first lumbar vertebrae in the adult, but in the infant it may reach as low as the third lumbar vertebra. Because of the disproportionate growth in length of the vertebral column during development, as compared with that of the spinal cord, the length of the spinal nerve roots increases progressively from above downwards. In the upper cervical regions, the spinal nerve roots are short and run almost horizontally, but the roots of the lumbar and sacral nerves below the level of the termination of the cord (lower border of the first lumbar vertebra in the adult and the lower border of the third lumbar vertebra in the infant) form a vertical leash of nerves known as the cauda equina. The spinal nerve supplying the reflex arcs for the knee and ankle jerks may therefore leave the vertebral column at a height of three to four vertebral bodies below the point at which the roots emanate from the spinal cord.

Abnormal reflexes

Increased tendon reflexes An abnormally brisk reflex is usually abnormal; unfortunately, an absent reflex is not usually absent but simply not elicited. Herein lies the major problem with testing children's reflexes. Always remember that the knee jerks are the easiest to elicit and the triceps the most difficult, and interpret your findings accordingly. Reflexes are rarely absent or pathologically brisk in the absence of other signs of neurological abnormality. Do not try to elicit a reflex while the child is moving that limb.

When tendon reflexes are pathologically increased, the contractions often spread beyond the stimulated muscle such as finger flexion, which often accompanies exaggerated upper limb reflexes.

Finger jerk (C7,8 and T1) (Fig. 7.13)
- Accompanies hyperreflexia
- Place the tips of your fingers over the palmar surface of the child's relaxed fingers. When you tap your own fingers, the child's fingers flex briskly.

Hoffman's sign (Fig. 7.14)
- Accompanies hyperreflexia
- Stabilize the child's middle phalanx between your first finger and thumb. Then flick the distal interphalangeal joint with your middle finger. If the tendon reflexes are hyperactive, the thumb will flex.

Primitive reflexes These are lost, or altered, as development progresses. The following reflexes disappear in 95% by the time specified:

- palmar grasp – 4 months
- stepping reflex – 4 months
- rooting reflex – 4 months

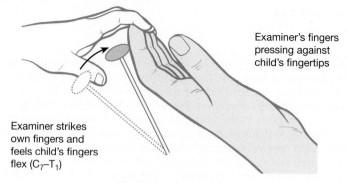

Examiner's fingers pressing against child's fingertips

Examiner strikes own fingers and feels child's fingers flex (C_7–T_1)

Fig. 7.13 Finger jerks.

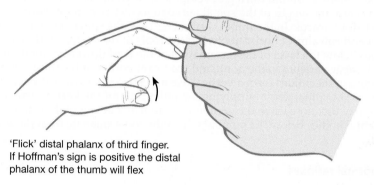

'Flick' distal phalanx of third finger. If Hoffman's sign is positive the distal phalanx of the thumb will flex

Fig. 7.14 Hoffman's sign.

- traction response – 4 months
- primary supporting – 6 months
- Moro reflex – 6 months
- crossed extensors – 6 months
- asymmetric tonic neck reflex – 6 months
- upgoing plantar – 12 months
- Galant response (scratch along a paravertebral line, the spine curves in with concavity on the stimulated side) – 5 years.

Persistence of these primitive reflexes beyond these age limits reflects failure of the CNS to mature. An extensor plantar response after 1 year of age implies an upper motor neurone lesion in the pyramidal tracts of brain or cord.

NEUROLOGICAL EXAMINATION OF THE OLDER CHILD

Neurological cases commonly seen in the MRCPCH or DCH in this age group are:

- hydrocephalus
- cerebral palsy
- cerebellar signs
- children who have had meningitis or an encephalopathy with residual abnormalities

- tuberous sclerosis
- spinal cord pathologies
- neurofibromatosis type I
- Guillain–Barré syndrome
- children who have had neurosurgery.

The comments on general inspection apply as for the younger child. The essence of examining the nervous system of a cooperative child is to have a well-rehearsed system of simple commands, which are unambiguous for the child, and interpretable responses.

INSPECTION

Inspect as for the infant:

- overall size and proportions of head/trunk/limbs
- dysmorphic features
- posture
- movement – gross and fine movement, sitting and standing:
  — general paucity
  — asymmetry
  — accessory.

CRANIAL NERVES (see pp. 125–143)

ARMS

When examining the limbs always examine the normal side first. Undress the child to the waist.

Inspection
Ask the child to stand with arms outstretched, fingers as wide apart as possible and tongue out. Look for:

- wasting
  — proximally > distally in muscular dystrophies and myopathies
  — distally > proximally in neuropathies
  — simultaneous wasting and pseudohypertrophy of different muscle groups in Duchenne's muscular dystrophy
- fasciculation
- involuntary movements
- asymmetry – 'Which hand do you write with?'; 'Stretch out your arms and play the piano' (demonstrating the action yourself). This will give you an idea of any gross asymmetry between the upper limbs before you begin more detailed assessment.

Tone
Always ask the child: 'Would it hurt if I were to move your arm?' Passively flex and extend the elbow and the wrist; spasticity is easier to detect than decreased tone. Children find it very difficult to relax but you can 'fool' them by rapid pronation/supination at the wrist or, for example, by asking them what they had for breakfast while you are assessing tone. Increased range of movement about joints is a frequent adjunct to hypotonia but do not confuse these two signs. Repeat with the opposite arm.

Power

Many candidates end up confusing the child and themselves when they attempt to test the child's power. The crucial points are:

● Have a simple system rather than an exhaustive one. Test the power of movement of major joints.
● First demonstrate what action you want the child to make, using your own hand or arm.
● Put the child's arm in the position you want to test and then get him/her to push against you.

Table 7.4 describes an approach to testing the power of a child's arms. This simple screen will detect most causes of weakness in the upper limbs. More detailed testing will result in both the child and the examiners losing concentration and is not worthwhile as isolated muscle and peripheral nerve lesions are rare in childhood.

Power may be recorded quantitatively using the grading recommendations by the Medical Research Council, i.e.:

0 – no contraction
1 – flicker of contraction
2 – active movement, with gravity eliminated (often difficult to test)
3 – active movement against gravity
4 – movement against resistance
5 – normal power.

However, you are only likely to be expected to say whether power is normal, reduced or absent.

Reflexes

Test these as described for younger children. Reflexes will be absent, normal or increased; some children have quite brisk reflexes but if there are no other signs of upper motor neurone weakness, assume the reflexes are normal. If you cannot elicit the reflexes, but there are no other signs of lower motor neurone or muscle weakness, try 'reinforcing' the jerk. Tendon reflexes are increased in amplitude by forcible contraction of muscles remote from those being tested.

Table 7.4 Testing the power of the arms

Request	Movement	Innervation
Place the child's arms so that they are about 45° away from the body		
'Push your elbows away from your body'	Shoulder abduction	C5
'Pull your elbows into your body'	Shoulder adduction	C6,7,8
Bend the child's arm so that the elbow is at a right angle		
'Pull me towards you'	Elbow flexion	C5,6
'Now try and straighten your arm'	Elbow extension	C7,8
Ask the child to make a fist		
'Don't let me bend your wrist'	Wrist flexion/extension	C6,7
Ask the child to spread the fingers		
'Don't let me squeeze them together'	Finger abduction	T1

Jendrassik's manoeuvre Demonstrate that you want the child to screw up his/her face (or pull the hands against each other if testing reflexes in the legs) on your command. The crucial point is that you must get the child do this just before you strike the tendon; otherwise the reinforcing effect will be lost.

Coordination

This is a composite function requiring normal motor, sensory and cerebellar systems and there is a very wide range among normal children. Again, therefore, do not make too much of these tests unless supported by other abnormal signs.

Finger–nose test Instruct the child as follows: 'Stretch your arm right out and touch my finger with your fingertip. Now touch your nose and then my finger and keep going until I say stop.' You may actually have to take hold of the child's finger and demonstrate what to do a few times (Fig. 7.15).

The test has not been performed correctly unless the movements are executed fairly quickly and you move your finger around in the field of vision (this test of coordination also requires normal vision) to provide a different target each time.

You are looking for intention tremor (the child's hand oscillates as it approaches the target) and past pointing (the hand overshoots or simply misses the target), both signs of cerebellar disease.

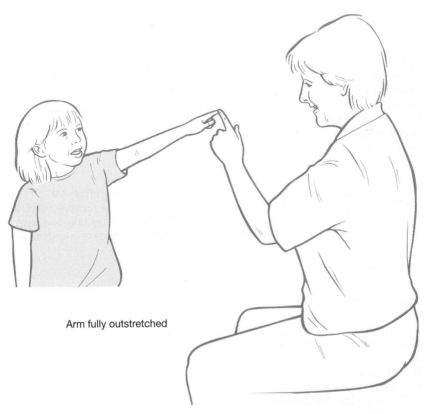

Arm fully outstretched

Fig. 7.15 Finger–nose test.

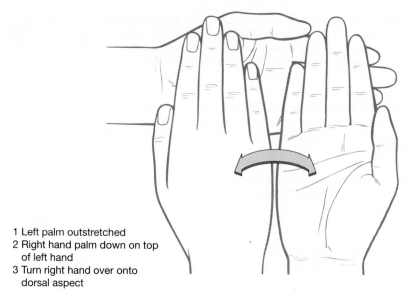

1 Left palm outstretched
2 Right hand palm down on top
  of left hand
3 Turn right hand over onto
  dorsal aspect

Fig. 7.16   Testing for dysdiadochokinesis.

Testing for dysdiadochokinesis   Dysdiadochokinesis is impairment of
rapid alternating movements.

Show the child that you want him/her to tap one hand with the other,
alternately tapping with the palm and back of the hand (Fig. 7.16). Other
examples of rapidly alternating actions are to mimic piano playing and to
touch the fingers of the hand alternately with the thumb of the same hand.
Children are always markedly better at these sorts of tasks with their
dominant hand and you must allow for this. Slowness and clumsiness at such
tasks are classically attributed to cerebellar disease but we must emphasize
that abnormalities of tone or power in that limb will produce similar
difficulties. Diadochokinesia should be smooth and rapid by the age of 8 years.

Look for overflow movements in the other hand.

Writing and drawing   These activities require enormous efforts of
coordination, of course, but as you will not have a baseline for that child, as
there is such wide variation with age and ability, and as they take too long
for the short cases, we would not advise using these as tests of coordination.

Sensation (Fig. 7.17)

Testing of the sensory modalities can be performed as follows:

- light touch – cotton wool
- superficial pain – pin prick
- deep pain – tendon reflexes
- temperature – warm/cold
- proprioception – joint position
- vibration – tuning fork
- cortical localization
  — two-point discrimination
  — stereognosis
  — graphaesthesia.

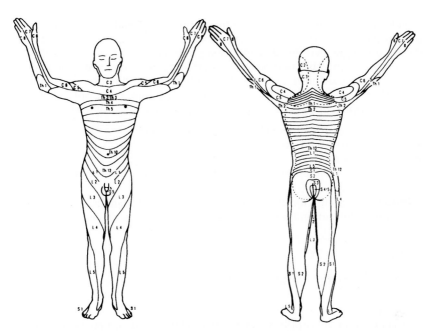

Fig. 7.17 Sensory dermatomes. (Reproduced with permission from Diem K, Lentner C (eds) 1970 Geigy-Scientific Tables, 7th edn. Ciba-Geigy, Basle.)

You are unlikely to be asked to test sensation in a short case but you would be expected to do this for a neurological long case. Do not test for pain or temperature sensation unless you are considering syringomyelia (lower motor neurone weakness in the arms, spasticity in the legs, possibly an associated spina bifida or sacral naevus) in which case there is loss of pain and temperature sensation in a cape distribution with light touch and proprioception unaffected ('dissociated sensory loss').

Light touch   Use a wisp of cotton wool and demonstrate the sensation this will cause. Ask the child to close his/her eyes and to say 'yes' immediately your touch is felt. Touch the skin lightly at each of the following sites (do not rub the cotton wool along the skin):

● lateral surface upper arm	C5
● tip of thumb	C6
● web between index and middle fingers	C7
● tip of little finger	C8
● medial surface lower arm	T1
● medial surface upper arm	T2

This simple method of sensory testing, in which the child is only expected to say 'yes' if touched, avoids some of the subjectivity and poor reproducibility for which testing sensation in children is notorious. There should be no delay in the child's response and you should only accept an unequivocal 'yes'.

Proprioception   Children enjoy this game. Hold the middle phalanx of the child's index finger and flex and extend the distal phalanx, telling the child which direction you mean by up and down. Now ask the child to close his/her eyes and say 'up' or 'down' when you move the finger. Remember to hold the distal phalanx by the sides, not the pulp, and not to follow any regular pattern. Start with fairly large excursions to convince yourself that the child has grasped the idea and then gradually reduce the size of the movement. Remember that normal proprioception is very sensitive and a normal child will detect movements of only a few millimetres. Try it out! It is worth testing only index finger and great toe joints, as the only likely cause of proprioceptive loss in a child is a peripheral neuropathy:

● vincristine neuropathy in children with leukaemia
● Guillain–Barré syndrome
● Friedreich's ataxia
● Charcot–Marie–Tooth disease and other hereditary neuropathies.

Vibration Testing vibration sense in children is difficult and unlikely to give more information than the above.

LEGS

Expose the legs from the groin downwards.

Inspection
The same comments apply as for younger children. If you are only asked to examine the child's legs, ensure that you make a brief general inspection of the child's face for any clues such as dysmorphic features, myopathy or drooling. Look for:

● muscle wasting
● asymmetry
● foot drop
● deformity.

Always look at the gait before formally examining the child's legs on the bed.
   Width of gait
● Normal children >3 years – 10–20 cm
● Very narrow gait – adductor spasm of a mild diplegia
● Wide gait
   — weakness or hypotonia of legs or pelvic girdle
   — cerebellar dysfunction
   — problems at the hip joint.
   Tests of gait
● By 3 years
   — walk on his/her heels and tip-toes
   — run
   — stand on one leg for 5 seconds
● By 4 years – able to hop
● By 5 years – able to walk in a straight line for 20 steps
● By 7 years – tandem walking (heel–toe walking).

At this stage it is worth asking the child to crouch down and then to stand up. This will quickly assess the strength of the distal and proximal muscles, respectively.

If there is persistent deviation or swaying, there may be abnormalities of tone, cerebellar dysfunction or a sensory neuropathy. If there are excessive associated movements of the arms, or clenching of the fists, particularly in a child over 8, the development of balance is slow.

Gaits which are uncommon in toddlers but occur in the older age group are:

- foot drop – peroneal muscular atrophy
- dystonic gait – the effort of walking may exacerbate the slow, writhing movements of athetoid cerebral palsy, Wilson's disease and torsion dystonia.

Foot deformities and their recognized associations are discussed in the chapter on examination of the joints (Ch. 10, The musculoskeletal system).

Tone

Test this as for the younger child. Remember to distract the child by talking to him/her. Cerebral palsy is still the commonest cause of spasticity in the legs in this age group but brain tumours and cord problems are more common than in infants.

Power

Again you need a very simple set of commands to test the necessary minimum of muscle groups (see Table 7.5). Say to the child: 'I'm going to test how strong you are.' You must oppose the child's actions; children enjoy this 'test of strength' and will exert themselves fully.

We have given the root levels for each of the actions in Table 7.5. It is not worth learning the actual muscle or nerve responsible for each of these actions as isolated lesions are very rare. Remember that pyramidal weakness (upper motor neurone lesion) causes more pronounced weakness in the extensors of the arm and in the flexors of the leg, and the weakness affects movements rather than individual muscles.

- *Cortical lesions* cause contralateral paralysis, a discrete lesion in the motor cortex giving rise to a circumscribed weakness.
- *A lesion in the internal capsule* usually causes a complete contralateral hemiparesis as the descending fibres are grouped close together.
- *Brain stem lesions* often affect both sides.

Table 7.5 Testing the power of the legs

Request	Movement	Innervation
'Lift your leg off the bed and keep it there; don't let me push it down'	Hip flexion	L1,2
'Push your leg into the bed; don't let me lift it off the bed'	Hip extension	L5,S1
'Bend your knee; now try to straighten your leg out as if you are kicking me away'	Knee extension	L3,4
'Bend your knee and try to pull your heel up towards your bottom'	Knee flexion	S1
'Pull your toes up towards your head'	Plantar flexion	L4,5
'Pull your big toe up towards your head'		L,5
'Point your toes towards the bed'	Plantar extension	S1,2
'Turn your foot inwards'	Foot inversion	L4,5
'Turn your foot outwards'	Foot eversion	L5,S1

● *A lesion in the spinal cord* gives an ipsilateral spastic paralysis below the lesion, possibly with lower motor neurone signs at the level of the lesion. Also look for sensory signs of bladder/bowel involvement.

Reflexes

These are elicited as for the younger child, possibly with the help of reinforcement, e.g. Jendrassik's maneouvre. This time ask the child to pull one hand against the other just before you strike the tendons with the hammer. Always watch that the head is central when testing reflexes, as the briskness of reflexes may be increased on the side to which the face is turned by the asymmetric tonic neck reflex. Children tend to have brisker reflexes in the legs than in the arms. Absence of the ankle jerks only may be the first evidence of a peripheral neuropathy, while preservation of the ankle jerks and absence of the knee jerks is more common in myopathies.

The Babinski response This test may be very uncomfortable for a child. The correct method is to start near the heel, and to stroke (not gouge) your finger or an orange stick (not a key) along the lateral aspect of the sole and then medially across the ball of the foot. Splaying of the toes and dorsiflexion of the big toe are indicative of a positive response. This implies there is an upper motor neurone lesion but tells you nothing about the level of this lesion. Usually, however, the response is one of withdrawal of the foot from this unpleasant stimulus, in which case the test is uninformative (not equivocal) and there is no point in repeating it several times to the anguish of the child and the examiners.

Testing of abdominal reflexes (T7–T12) and cremaster reflex (L1, 2) is not a routine part of the examination. If you are trying to establish the level of a cord lesion, look for a sensory level for light touch.

Clonus Sustained clonus is evidence of an upper motor neurone lesion, although one or two beats, in the absence of any other signs, may be ignored. Ankle clonus may be obtained by rapidly dorsiflexing the ankle and patellar clonus by pushing the patella downwards with the knee straight.

Coordination

If gait, tone and power are normal, tests of coordination in the legs are so gross as to be a waste of time. Likewise, if gait, tone and power are abnormal, tests of coordination will not tell you anything new, but for completeness, include the heel–shin test.

Heel–shin test Ask the child to place one heel on the top of the opposite knee and then to slide the heel down the front of the shin to the ankle and back up to the knee. Ask the child to repeat the maneouvre several times steadily and accurately as rapidly as possible.

Sensation (see Fig. 7.17)

As for the arms, test only light touch and joint position sense.
Anteriorly
● Inguinal region   L1
● Medial surface of upper thigh   L2
● Medial surface of lower thigh   L3
● Medial surface of lower leg   L4
● Lateral surface of lower leg   L5
● Lateral surface of foot   S1

Posteriorly
- Medial surface of upper calf   S2
- Medial surface of inner thigh   S3
- Perianal surface   S4

Only test perineal sensation if there is other evidence of a sacral cord or cauda equina lesion. The perianal skin is supplied by S3, 4, 5 and the anal sphincter may appear lax ('S2, 3, 4 keeps the faeces off the floor') or there may be obvious incontinence.

LIMB GIRDLE AND TRUNK

The ability to test these muscle groups in children is important as the muscular dystrophies present with proximal muscle weakness. Often the initial complaint is of problems with walking, running or climbing stairs. Apart from formal testing of shoulder movements and straight leg raising as outlined above, the following may be helpful.

The shoulder girdle
Ask the child to mime combing of the hair. He/she may be able to do this initially but will tire quickly.

The trunk
Can the child sit up from a supine position without the aid of the arms?

The pelvic girdle
Standing from a crouching position requires powerful proximal muscles. Ask the child to do the following: 'Kneel down on the floor; now stand up without using your hands.'

Gower's sign
This describes a manoeuvre used to get up off the floor, first described in boys with Duchenne's muscular dystrophy. Instruct as follows: 'Lie on your back; now try to stand up without using your hands.' The child will roll onto the front and then push against the thighs to straighten up, effectively *climbing up his/her legs.*

CEREBELLAR SYSTEM

The cerebellar system is involved in coordination of movements and dysfunction leads to incoordinate, imprecise movements rather than weakness. The features may occasionally be associated with hypotonia and hyporeflexia. Most of the features have been described in previous sections but it is helpful to have a structured routine just for cerebellar examination, in order to ensure that you are not thrown if such a request is made in the exam (see Table 7.6). The posterior fossa is the commonest site of childhood brain tumours.

Romberg's sign
If there is evidence of ataxia, test for Romberg's sign, which provides evidence of ataxia due to proprioceptive sensory loss; rare in childhood.

Table 7.6 Examining the cerebellar system

Request	Abnormality
Chat to the child to assess speech *'Hello, what is your name?'*	'Scanning' dysarthria
'Look straight ahead at me' – are the eyes steady?	Nystagmus
Show the child that you want him/her to tap one hand with the other, alternately tapping with the palm and back of the hand (see Fig. 7.16). Remember, the non-dominant hand is always slower	Dysdiadochokinesis
'Reach out and touch my finger' – the child's hand is steady at rest but develops a tremor of increasing amplitude as it approaches the target	Intention tremor
The child will overshoot the target when reaching out to touch it	Dysmetria
'Pretend you are in the circus and walking along a tightrope' – the candidate should demonstrate heel-to-toe walking	Ataxic gait

The child stands with the feet together. Observe for a few seconds and then ask the child to close his/her eyes. The sign is positive if the child is significantly more unsteady without visual cues.

HIGHER FUNCTION

Tests of memory and concentration are difficult in children because of the wide variation between individuals and with age. It is more sensible to be guided by the parents and by changes in school performance (provided vision and hearing are known to be normal). However, if a child has a hemiparesis, you should know how to test some higher cortical functions.

INSPECTION

- Appearance, e.g. any dysmorphism, obvious hemiparesis
- Behaviour, e.g. bewildered, restless, agitated
- Emotional state, e.g. laughing inappropriately in Angelman's syndrome.

CONSCIOUS LEVEL

Although it is unlikely you will encounter a patient who is not fully conscious in the exam, you may be asked how to assess consciousness in a young child and you should be familiar with the Glasgow Coma Scale for children (see p. 24).

SPEECH

This can be crudely assessed from general conversation with the child. This section is not intended to be a comprehensive section on speech assessment. We have omitted receptive dysphasia, mutism and autism, etc., which are unlikely cases in the exam, and assessment of which is outwith the confines of this book.

Expressive dysphasia This is easily tested by asking the child to name simple objects such as a pen, watch, etc. You can check that the child's vocabulary is adequate and that it is a purely expressive problem by demonstrating to the examiners that, while unable to name them, he/she can still point to the pen and watch.

Sensory perception There may be right/left discrimination problems or gross sensory inattention for the contralateral visual field or side of the body. More subtle disturbance may be shown by testing graphaesthesia; ask the child to close his/her eyes and say what number you are drawing on the palm of his/her hand. Draw slowly, making clear strokes.

If the child has had a hemiplegia since birth due to cerebral palsy, these tests may be normal as the brain has had time to adapt. However, if the problem is recent or if the onset was after the pre-school years, parietal function may be abnormal.

Always remember to measure and plot head circumference. If the child's head is abnormally large or small, also measure and plot the parents' head circumference.

COMMON NEUROLOGICAL LONG CASES

CEREBRAL PALSY

Candidates who score badly on this case do so either because they fail to take an appropriate history or because they have little practical experience of the outpatient approach to long-term management. The physical signs are usually obvious and rarely missed although they may be demonstrated poorly.

Cerebral palsy (CP) is a motor disorder as a result of non-progressive brain damage in early life, with a prevalence of 2.5 per 1000 children. Although it is a disorder of motor function, damage to other parts of the brain can be expected to a greater or lesser extent, including speech disorders, learning difficulties, hearing and visual problems and epilepsy. Classification of cerebral palsy centres around the motor manifestations of brain damage, which can be due to malfunctioning of the cerebral cortex (spasticity), the cerebellum (ataxia) and the basal ganglia (dyskinesia). Over the past few decades it has become increasingly apparent that an underlying cause exists. Improved imaging techniques enable confirmation that most children with hemiplegia have sustained an antenatal stroke. With advances in perinatal care, the aetiology of cerbral palsy is also changing. Choreoathetoid cerebral palsy associated with kernicterus is no longer seen. Improvements in obstetric management have reduced the incidence of birth trauma and intrapartum asphyxia. In contrast, cerbral palsy secondary to intraventricular haemorrhage is increasing as more very low birthweight babies are surviving.

HISTORY

The history must address:

● possible causes
● the impact of this disorder on the child and family
● the steps taken to minimize the effects of the disorder.

169

Obstetric and perinatal history

The aetiology of cerebral palsy may be prenatal, perinatal or postnatal; therefore, enquire about:

- infection and infectious contacts during pregnancy
- concern from ultrasound scans about the baby's growth
- vaginal bleeding during pregnancy
- high blood pressure and ankle swelling
- diabetes
- a detailed history of the labour and mode of delivery; how many weeks pregnant?
- whether forceps or caesarean section were necessary; if so, does the mother know why?
- whether a paediatrician was present at the delivery
- birthweight
- fetal movements.

If the infant was admitted to the special care baby unit, then clearly a detailed account of the infant's problems, treatment and length of stay is required. In particular, ask about:

- whether a breathing machine was necessary
- neonatal encephalopathy
- seizures
- brain scans
- exchange transfusion for jaundice
- neonatal meningitis.

Remember, in the vast majority of cases of CP, a term infant was born by a normal delivery following a perfectly healthy pregnancy.

Presentation

The commonest characteristics are:

- abnormal tone and posturing in early infancy
- delayed motor milestones noted by the parents
- a floppy baby, or alternatively increased tone. Hypotonia often precedes the development of spasticity
- feeding problems
- delayed acquisition of language and social skills
- irritability
- seizures
- motor delay or asymmetry detected incidentally at routine screening, or at follow-up of some other problem such as deafness or visual loss.

Most children with CP are not diagnosed definitely until after the first year of life, but often some of the above features are apparent in retrospect. Many candidates mistakenly think that most cases of CP derive from the population of premature infants. In fact, less than 25% of cases have been born prematurely and although most centres closely follow all 'at risk' premature infants, most are entirely normal. A particular subgroup of CP, spastic diplegia, does however have an association with low birthweight.

Developmental history

Only the motor milestones may have been delayed but often there are other associated problems (see below).

Family history
Are there any relatives with physical or mental handicap or neurological disease with the onset in early childhood?

Associated non-motor problems
These are common and may represent more of a handicap to the child than the motor disorder itself.

- Visual impairment from refraction errors or cortical damage – 20%
- Squints – 30%
- Hearing impairment (usually sensorineural) – 20%
- Epilepsy – 40%
- Moderate learning difficulties (IQ 50–70) – 30%
- Severe learning difficulties (IQ <50) – 30%
- Speech and language disorders
- Behaviour disorders.

Therefore, ask specifically about:

- sight, squints and spectacles
- hearing and hearing aids
- speech
- mobility
- deformity
- continence and constipation
- feeding problems
- seizures and anticonvulsant medication
- behaviour problems
- recurrent chest infections.

It is a mistake to assume that the degree of physical and mental handicap go hand-in-hand.

Special aids
- Does the child have any special aids to help compensate for the handicap:
  — glasses
  — hearing aid
  — splints
  — special shoes
  — wheelchair
  — communication aids?
- Have any special modifications been made to the house, in particular to the toilet and bathroom or to accommodate a wheelchair? An extension may have been necessary, or even a move to a new house.

Education
The needs of the child will be different at different ages and you need to have an understanding of who caters for these needs and how they are catered for. There is a change from a predominantly health-led multidisciplinary team approach in the pre-school child to an educational authority child-development team approach in the school-age child. Attending to the educational needs of the child is a crucial part of long-term management. If the child attends a special school, some of the therapists already mentioned may be on the staff or attend regularly. However, since the Warnock report, children are encouraged to attend normal schools, especially if their handicap is purely physical. A nursery

nurse may be assigned to the class to provide extra support for the child. If the child does have learning difficulties, an educational psychologist will also be involved.

Sources of help to the family

What other sources of help do the parents have, financial or otherwise? Ask about:

- local self-help groups, charities and relatives
- arrangements for 'respite care' to allow the parents time for a holiday and more time with the child's siblings
- are they entitled to claim an attendance allowance (possible for children over 2 years of age) or a mobility allowance (for children over 5 years of age)?

Effect on family members

Ask about the effect of the child's handicap on other members of the family, especially siblings.

Medication

Ask about:

- regular medications (anticonvulsants, antispasmodics, night sedation)
- nutritional supplements.

Finally, despite all these problems, try not to lose sight of what the child can do, rather than concentrating only on what he/she cannot do, e.g. the simple activities of daily living: dressing, toileting, feeding. There are probably particular games or sports which the child prefers, in which the physical disability is less of a handicap, especially swimming. This functional assessment is not the same as a developmental or neurological assessment.

MANAGEMENT

A multidisciplinary team approach is fundamental to the management of a child with cerebral palsy. Ask in detail about the input of the professionals listed below – how often does the child see them, what exactly do they do, and do the parents feel that the child derives any benefit?

- General practitioner
- Paediatrician
- Optician and ophthalmologist
- Orthopaedic surgeon
- Health visitor
- Community nurse
- Physiotherapist
- Occupational therapist
- Speech and language therapist
- Educational psychologist
- Social workers
- Teachers.

EXAMINATION

The aims are to define the following.

The type of CP

Spastic (70%)
- Hemiplegia – usually arm > leg
- Quadriplegia ('double hemiplegia') – arms > legs
- Diplegia – legs > arms.
  Ataxic (10%)
  Dyskinetic (10%)
- Monoplegic
- Dystonic
- Choreoid
- Athetoid
- Mixed.

The severity
This is defined in terms of how the disability affects the child's ability to function, emphasizing what the child can rather than cannot do.

Associated disabilities
A full neurological examination should be performed but particular attention should be paid to the following:

Posture
- Arm flexed, fisting, and leg extended in hemiplegia
- Scissoring of spastic diplegia – when standing, the child's body is tilted forward and the hips and knees flexed; when sitting, the back is arched
- Windswept (gravitational) posture of a very inactive child.

Tone
- Increased in 70% of cases
- This clasp-knife spasticity is classically demonstrated by extending the elbow and stretching biceps but may be much more obvious on supination of the wrist. It is a velocity-related increase in tone with passive stretch.
- The child may have been hypotonic initially
- In atonic CP, reflexes are normal or increased.

Power There may be abnormalities of tone and reflexes without obvious loss of power. However, there may then be a reduction of voluntary movements and obvious premature hand preference or exertion may precipitate an excess of involuntary, associated movements.

If power is severely reduced, contractures (or scars where they have been released) may be apparent and there may be trophic changes of dwarfing of the limb with cool, cyanosed or puffy skin.

Reflexes Brisk tendon jerks, clonus and extensor plantars may all occur in the spastic group.

Gait
Hemiplegia Look for:

- the child walking on the toes of the affected side
- extension of the knee and circumduction of the leg
- shortening of the Achilles tendon and occasionally clawing of the toes.

Cerebral diplegia   The child walks with hips and knees flexed, taking the weight on the toes. Steps are short and rotation of the body may be used to advance the leading foot.

Ataxic CP   A broad-based gait with arms raised to improve balance.

Cerebellar function   10% of CP is of the ataxic type. Look for:

● hypotonia
● paucity of spontaneous movements
● resting tremor of head and intention tremor of hand, e.g. ask the child to hold a cup
● nystagmus – very rare unless there is an associated visual problem.

Involuntary movements   Athetosis is the commonest form of dyskinesia in CP, but chorea, tremor and truncal dystonia also occur. Pharyngeal incoordination often leads to drooling and dysarthria. There may be associated extensor spasms and yet hypotonia, but not weakness, is very common in this group. Contractures are rare.

DISCUSSION POINTS

● You must be able to discuss the multidisciplinary team approach to managing these patients.
● The impact of coping with a child with a chronic disease can be a significant burden on the family, and examiners like to discuss the social and emotional implications for the family. Familiarity with financial benefits and support for the family will be expected.
● Moves away from schools for children with special needs towards integration into mainstream schools provides a topic for debate on the relative merits of each type of education system.
● You must be aware of the new treatments available for spasticity, in particular baclofen and botulinum toxin. Oral medication is not well tolerated, with only minimal efficacy. Multicentre studies on intrathecal baclofen infusions have demonstrated its effectiveness in decreasing spasticity associated with cerebral palsy. However, adverse side-effects, such as nausea and vomiting, hypotonia and seizures (in patients with established epilepsy), are reported in a significant number of patients.
● Botulinum toxin type A is increasingly being used for the treatment of spasticity in children with cerebral palsy. Botulinum injections have been successfully used to reduce the equinus deformity associated with tight peroneal muscles. However, it should be stressed that such treatments should be used with adjuvant physiotherapy, orthosis and casting.

COMMON NEUROLOGICAL SHORT CASES

● The floppy infant
● Small head
● Large head
● The child in a wheelchair
● Examination of the legs
● Mixed upper and lower motor neurone signs.

All young babies are floppy to a certain degree so a quantitative assessment of whether the hypotonia is pathological is required. Floppiness may be associated with weakness, muscular in origin, or with no associated muscle weakness, central in origin. In the majority of cases, the hypotonia is cerebral in origin.

Neuromuscular disease is suggested by hypotonia accompanied by weakness, suggested by:

- paucity of movements
- a weak cry
- a poor suck
- hypoventilation and possibly paradoxical respiration (chest wall muscles weaker than diaphragm) or chest deformity, classically bell-shaped
- muscle wasting and winging of the scapula.

Causes of hypotonia

Central
- Down's syndrome
- Cerebral palsy (in addition to these two common causes of hypotonia, many other conditions in which mental retardation occurs are associated with hypotonia)
- Hypothyroidism
- Prader–Willi syndrome
- Some storage disorders (e.g. Niemann–Pick disease, infantile Tay–Sachs disease).

Nerve or muscle weakness   Classify anatomically:
  Anterior horn cell
- Spinal muscular atrophy
- Myelomeningocele
- Traumatic or asphyxial cord lesions
- Poliomyelitis.
  Peripheral nerve
- Guillain–Barré syndrome
- Lead poisoning.
  Neuromuscular junction
- Myasthenia gravis.
  Muscle
- Simple failure to thrive
- The muscular dystrophies
- Dystrophia myotonica
- Acid maltase deficiency (Pompé's disease)
- Congenital myopathies (nemaline rod, central core, etc.).

Genuine hypotonia should not be confused with increased joint laxity but both may be encountered simultaneously in conditions such as:

- osteogenesis imperfecta
- Ehlers–Danlos syndrome
- Marfan's syndrome.

EXAMINATION

Posture
- Characteristic 'frog's legs'.

Face
- Dysmorphism
  — any obvious syndrome?
  — shake hands with the parent (inability to relax grip in dystrophia myotonica)
- Tongue fasciculation suggests spinal muscular atrophy
- Protruding tongue suggests Down's syndrome, hypothyroidism or Pompé's disease
- A child who is alert and interested is unlikely to have one of the conditions associated with mental retardation
- The presence of a nasogastric tube may be due to difficulties with sucking or swallowing (e.g. cerebral disorder as in infantile Batten's disease or bulbar palsy as in Werdnig–Hoffmann disease).

Lift the child
- Slips through your fingers
- Rag doll on ventral suspension
- Head lag on traction.

Formally assess tone, power and reflexes (as described previously)

Remember to look at the genitalia (small penis in Prader–Willi syndrome) **and the spine** (myelomeningocele)

SMALL HEAD

Head size is closely correlated with brain size but much more loosely with intelligence. Microcephaly is defined as OFC < 3rd centile.

Measurements
- Head circumference
- Height
- Weight
- Plot all three on an appropriate centile chart
- Measure the head circumference of all siblings and parents present.

NORMAL VARIATION

The proportionately small child may have a small head. If all measurements are more than three standard deviations away from the mean, consider causes of dwarfing (e.g. Russell–Silver syndrome).

FAMILIAL

Parents with small heads often have children with small heads despite normal length and weight.

PATHOLOGICAL

Genetic (also called primary microcephaly)

There is characteristic facies with sloping forehead and little brow; associated with mental retardation and may be an autosomal recessive inheritance. The brain is morphologically normal on CT scan.

Secondary microcephaly

Perinatal insult   The face looks normal.
- Congenital infection – look for hepatosplenomegaly, purpura, choroidoretinitis, deafness, heart murmur
- Perinatal brain injury – normal OFC at birth but head size then falls away from the centiles. Hemiatrophy of the face or limbs may follow if the cerebral atrophy is unilateral.

Fetal alcohol syndrome
Syndromes with mental retardation
- Cornelia de Lange syndrome
- Rubinstein–Taybi syndrome
- Smith–Lemli–Opitz syndrome.

Syndromes with premature fusion of cranial sutures
- Apert's syndrome
- Crouzon's syndrome.

Infant of mother with phenylketonuria

LARGE HEAD

Measurements
- Head circumference
- Height
- Weight
- Plot all three on an appropriate centile chart
- Measure the head circumference of all the siblings and parents present.

The aetiologies of macrocephaly are usually divided into normotensive and hypertensive (look for signs of raised intracranial pressure, such as bulging fontanelle, distended scalp veins, sun-setting of eyes) since this distinction determines the urgency of investigation and treatment.

NORMOTENSIVE

Large brain (megalencephaly)

Anatomical megalencephaly: excessive growth
- Normal variants – a proportionately large baby with a large head, or a familial trait; the parents also have large heads
- Associated with dwarfism (e.g. achondroplasia) or gigantism (e.g. Soto's syndrome), and often developmental delay
- Neurofibromatosis.

Metabolic megalencephaly: storage diseases
- Maple syrup urine disease
- Mucopolysaccharidoses

- Alexander's disease
- Glutaric aciduria type I
- Canavan's disease.

Malformations
These may be accompanied by excessive head growth due to fluid accumulation.

- Hydranencephaly
- Porencephaly
- Holoprosencephaly.

Thickened calvarium of skull
Expansion of bone marrow
- Acquired or hereditary anaemia (classically thalassaemia).
Expansion of the bone itself
- Rickets
- Osteogenesis imperfecta
- Osteopetrosis
- Cleidocranial dysostosis.

HYPERTENSIVE

Chronic hydrocephalus
Communicating
- Previous periventricular, subarachnoid or subdural haemorrhage
- Previous meningitis
- Spina bifida with associated Arnold–Chiari malformation.
Non-communicating
- Congenital aqueduct stenosis
- Dandy–Walker syndrome
- Previous periventricular haemorrhage in a preterm infant
- Posterior fossa neoplasm.

Chronic cerebral oedema
- Benign intracranial hypertension
- Vitamin A intoxication.

Chronic subdural effusion
- Following birth trauma
- Following meningitis
- Following child abuse
- Menke's syndrome.

THE CHILD IN A WHEELCHAIR

The commonest causes are:

- Spina bifida – usually the lesion is above L2. The combination of talipes equinovarus, flexion contractures at the hip, urinary incontinence and a

patulous anus is virtually pathognomonic. The length and width of the lesion should be measured
- Duchenne's muscular dystrophy (by teenage)
- Cerebral palsy – 25% are unable to walk.

INSPECTION

- Overall posture – the use of foam or plastic wedges suggests that the child has difficulty in maintaining posture, often because of hypotonia
- Head size – hydrocephalus suggests spina bifida; palpate for shunt
- Face – any dysmorphic features?
- Shake hands with the child, if old enough, and ask him/her to propel the wheelchair forwards to assess power and function in the arms
- Indwelling urinary catheter and bag – again suggests spina bifida, or less commonly cord tumour or traumatic cord damage
- The presence of splints, supports, gaiters, calipers and specially adapted shoes may all hint at the sites of weakness or spasticity and should be commented on.

Do not attempt to examine the child in the wheelchair. Endeavour, with the aid of the parents, to help the child onto the bed, a task which provides much information about tone and mobility. If the examiners feel that this is unnecessary, they will tell you. Ensure that the child's legs are completely exposed whilst keeping the genitalia covered.

In the case of a child requiring a wheelchair, the crucial distinction to be made is whether the abnormality causing the paraparesis is:

- in the head
- in the cord
- peripheral nerve or muscle disease.

EXAMINATION OF THE LEGS

Candidates may be asked to 'examine the legs' of an ambulant child and the abnormal physical signs in this short case may not be neurological at all. A system for a complete examination of the lower limbs is as follows:

Exposure
- From the groin downwards.

Gait

Inspection
- Dysmorphic features
- Skin stigmata of neurological disease
- Asymmetry
- Scarring
- Deformity
- Trophic changes from denervation – shiny, cool skin with loss of hair, abnormal nail growth, possibly evidence of insensitivity to trauma
- Muscle wasting or contractures.

Feel

● For the femoral and foot pulses.

Joint examination

Ask if either limb hurts and, if not, progress to examine quickly each of the hip, knee and ankle joints for swelling or abnormal range of movement.

Neurological examination

If you have found no abnormalities so far, proceed to a formal neurological examination of the legs as described in the text – motor first and then sensory.

Spine and abdomen

Examine the spine and abdomen of a child with a paraparesis.

Anal tone

Offer to assess anal tone, although this will not be required in the exam.

MIXED UPPER AND LOWER MOTOR NEURONE SIGNS

The genuine combination of mixed upper and lower motor neurone signs is rare but candidates seem to find such signs with remarkable frequency and must be able to offer a few possible explanations:

● Cord damage at the C5–T1 level, irrespective of the cause (e.g. severe scoliosis, tumour, syringomyelia), may give rise to lower motor neurone signs in the arms and upper motor neurone signs in the legs.
● The following are childhood causes of mixed upper and lower motor neurone signs in the lower limbs:
   — *cord compression at L3/L4*: absent knee jerks and extensor plantar reflexes. Do not confuse cord compression with cauda equina compression, which causes lower motor neurone signs in the legs with 'saddle' sensory loss around the perineum and urinary incontinence
   — *'mixed' type of cerebral palsy*: various combinations of hypotonia and increased reflexes
   — *Friedreich's ataxia*: spasticity, extensor plantars, pes cavus and absent ankle reflexes
   — *metachromatic leucodystrophy*: spasticity and absent tendon reflexes
   — *vitamin B$_{12}$ deficiency*: spasticity, extensor plantars and absent ankle reflexes.

All except mixed cerebral palsy are rare, so consider carefully whether you have elicited the signs correctly.

A summary of the main sensory and motor pathways are shown in Figures 7.18 and 7.19.

The short cases are covered in more detail in *Paediatric Short Cases for Postgraduate Examinations* by A Thomson, H Wallace and T Stephenson (Churchill Livingstone, Edinburgh, 2003).

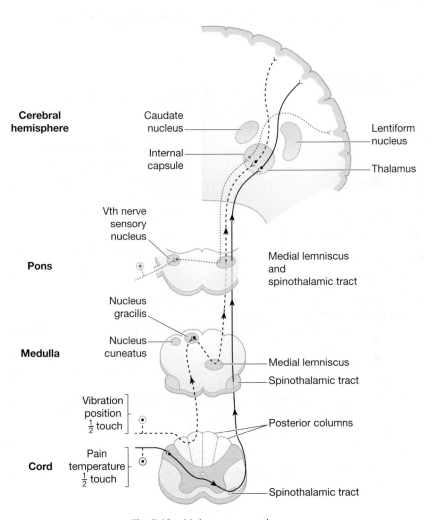

Fig. 7.18 Main sensory pathways.

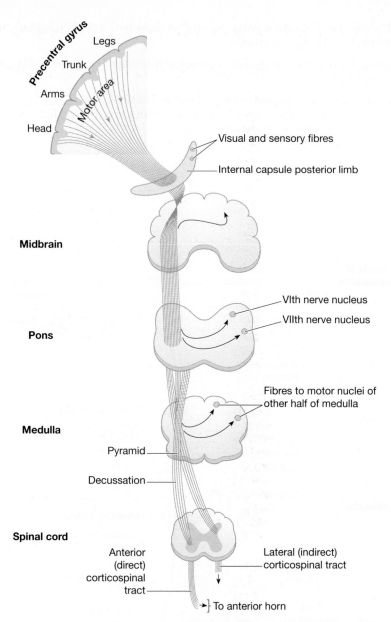

Fig. 7.19   Main motor pathways.

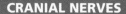

The nervous system

CRANIAL NERVES

Generally you will not be asked to examine all the cranial nerves in the exam but you you may be asked to examine any of the individual nerves or components.

I
Not directly tested. Can ask older child if there are any problems smelling food

II
Visual acuity
Need to know if the child can see and understand instructions. Begin with Snellen chart or print (for older child) and work down via counting fingers, detecting hand movement, distinguishing light from dark. The candidate who completely fails to realize a child is blind in one eye and progresses through a complex exam is not uncommon

Pupils
Direct and consensual light reflexes and accommodation reaction

Visual fields
Confrontation perimetry in older child – each eye in turn, then both. Younger child may need two examiners, one to distract and the other to bring a toy into the child's periphery from behind

Fundoscopy
Do at the end

III, IV, VI
Eye movements
'Follow my finger with your eyes' – holding the child's head still. 'Tell me if you can see two fingers at any point'

V
Motor
'Open your mouth and don't let me close it.' Feel masseters with teeth clenched (increased in Duchenne's muscular dystrophy)

Sensory
Test light touch in each of the three divisions. 'Close your eyes, say yes when you feel me touch you.' Is it the same on both sides?

VII
Motor
'Raise your eyebrows and screw your eyes up tight as if there is soap in them. Puff out your cheeks. Give me a big smile and show me your teeth.' Corneal reflex is not tested as too painful

Sensory
Supplies taste to anterior two-thirds of the tongue; seldom tested

VIII
Cochlear
Examine external auditory meati for local disease, wax, grommets.
Normal speech? In young infant lying down, you can clap or ring a bell and see if he/she turns head to sound. In sitting child use distraction hearing test

● Weber's test – 512-Hz tuning fork in centre of frontal bone:
— perceptive deafness: louder on healthy side
— conductive deafness: louder on diseased side
● Rinne's test – 512-Hz tuning fork placed on mastoid bone:
— conductive deafness: bone is louder
— perceptive deafness or normal hearing: air is louder

Vestibular
Nystagmus can be checked for when assessing eye movements

IX, X
'Gag reflex' – generally not tested but ask patient to say 'ah' and observe for symmetrical elevation of the palatal arches
Voice dysphonia. Swallowing intact
Sensation to posterior third of tongue, soft palate, nasopharynx (IX) not tested for

XI
'Can you shrug your shoulders?' – any muscle wasting?
'Turn your head against my hand to look over your shoulder'

XII
'Can you stick out your tongue?'

NEUROLOGICAL EXAMINATION OF A BABY/TODDLER

INSPECTION (fully dressed on parent's lap)
1. Overall size and proportions head/trunk/limbs
2. Dysmorphic features
3. Posture – asymmetrical – alarm bells
4. Movement – gross and fine movement, sitting/standing
   — general paucity
   — asymmetrical
   — accessory: tic, chorea, tremor, titubation, athetoid
   — convulsive

EYES
Start here as the child may cry
1. Eye-to-eye contact
2. Fixate?
3. Conjugate or squint?
4. Nystagmus/ptosis/cataract/iris/conjunctiva, etc.
5. Pupils
6. Test external occular movements with toy (fix and follow 180° by 4 months)

OTHER CRANIAL NERVES
VII – observe symmetry of smile
VII, IX, X, XII suck and swallow
VII, X, XII (speech)
Stammers are relatively common and unrelated to pathology
Delayed – learning difficulties, autism
   Difficult to understand (dysarthria much commoner than dysphasia) – cerebral palsy, speech disorder
Monotonous – deafness
XII – stick out tongue

HEAD
1. Shape
2. Sutures
3. Fontanelles
4. Size – measure OFC at end
5. Feel for VP shunt/reservoir

HANDS
1. Dysmorphic – syndactyly, polydactyly, clinodactyly, palmar creases
2. Muscle wasting
3. Handedness ($1\frac{1}{2}$ – 5 years); if <18 months think hemiplegia
4. Offer child a toy – does the child reach/grasp; is there any tremor; does the child transfer?

NOW UNDRESS TO NAPPY (if >3 years in nappy, ask why)
Simultaneously look for:
Muscle wasting
Scars for VP shunts, scoliosis, lower spine abnormalities

ARMS

Inspection
1. Deformity (bony and soft tissue, skin markings)
2. Muscle bulk
3. Posture

Tone
Increased = spasticity = UMNL = cerebral palsy in exams
Decreased/absent = LMNL/neuromuscular junction, muscle disorder

Power
Tightness of grasping object
Pull infant up by arms to supine

Coordination
Observe play, particularly watching the child's gait, manipulation of toys and ability to reach for toys

Reflexes
Increased in UMNL +/– clonus
Absent in LMNL

Sensation
Not done in exams unless indicated or specifically asked for.

TRUNK
Sit from supine and observe balance
Skin – abnormal skin markings suggesting TS of NF
Sacrum/spine

LEGS
Always start with **gait** – look for limp, broad-based, spastic, hemiplegic (circumduction and foot scuffs the floor), waddling, toe-walking
As for arms – inspection, tone, power, coordination and reflexes

NEUROLOGICAL EXAMINATION OF AN OLDER CHILD

INSPECTION (as for infant)
1. Overall size and proportions head/trunk/limbs
2. Dysmorphic features
3. Posture – asymmetrical – may indicate underlying pathology
4. Movement – gross and fine movement, sitting/standing
   — general paucity
   — asymmetrical
   — accessory: tic, chorea, tremor, titubation, athetoid
   — convulsive

ARMS
Undress to the waist

Inspection
'Hold your arms out straight like this' – look for wasting, fasciculation, involuntary movements
'Which hand do you write with?'
'Stretch out your arms and play the piano like this' – look for asymmetry

Always examine the normal side first

Tone
Ask if it would hurt to move the arm

Power
Ask the child to bend the arms and hold them up at 90° out to the side
C5 – shoulder abduction – 'Push your elbows away from your body'
C6,7,8 – shoulder adduction – 'Pull your elbows into your body'

Bend arms so that elbow is at right angle
C5,6 – elbow flexion – 'Pull me towards you'
C7,8 – elbow extension – 'Push me away'

Ask the child to make a fist
C6,7 – wrist flexion/extension – 'Don't let me bend your wrist'

Spread your fingers
T1 – finger abduction – 'Don't let me squeeze them together'

Reflexes
Use the Jendrassik manoeuvre if it is difficult to elicit the reflexes and there are no other abnormal signs. Demonstrate that you want the child to screw up his/her face (or to pull the hands against each other if testing leg reflexes) on your command, just before you strike the tendon

Coordination
Finger to nose touching
Dysdiadochokinesis – show the child that you want him/her to tap one hand with the other, alternately tapping the palm and the back of the hand

Sensation (not done unless requested)
Light touch
Proprioception

LEGS
Expose from groin downwards

Inspection
Also have a quick look at the child's face for any clues such as myopathy or drooling
Look for muscle wasting, asymmetry, limp, fasciculation, foot drop, deformity

Gait

By 3 years – walk on heels/tip-toes, run
  – stand on one leg for 5 seconds
By 4 years – hop
By 5 years – straight line for 20 steps
By 7 years – tandem walking (heel–toe walking)
  – fog test: child walks on lateral borders of feet and the hands are also noted to turn inwards – suggestive of cerebral lesion
Crouch down (distal muscles), now stand (proximal muscles)

Tone

Increased = spasticity = cerebral palsy

Power

'I'm going to test how strong you are'

L1,2	'Lift your leg off the bed; keep it there and don't let me push it down'
L5,S1	'Push your leg into the bed; don't let me lift it off the bed'
L3,4	'Bend your knee; now try to straighten your leg out as if you are kicking me'
S1	'Bend your knee and try to pull your heel up towards your bottom'
L4,5	'Pull your toes up towards your head'
L5	'Pull your big toe up towards your head'
S1,2	'Point your toes towards the bed'
L4,5	'Turn your foot inwards'
L5,S1	'Turn your foot outwards'

Reflexes

Remember reinforcement with Jendrassik's manoeuvre

Coordination

Heel–shin test

Sensation

Light touch
L1 – inguinal ligament
L2 – middle of anterior thigh
L3 – medial aspect of knee
L4 – medial calf
L5 – lateral calf
S1 – sole of foot
S3,4,5 – perineal sensation (don't test unless you suspect an abnormality)

ANYTHING ELSE?

Spine, head (posterior fossa scar), joints

NEUROLOGICAL EXAMINATION OF LIMB GIRDLE AND TRUNK (OLDER CHILD)

MUSCULAR DYSTROPHIES

Test shoulder movements
Straight leg raising

Shoulder Girdle

'Show me how you would comb your hair'

Trunk

'Can you lie on your back and sit up without using your hands?'

Pelvic girdle

'Kneel down on the floor. Now stand up without using your hands'

Gower's sign

'Lie on your back. Now try to stand up without using your hands.' Child rolls onto the front and then pushes up against his/her legs to get up, i.e. 'climbing up his legs'

187

Clinical paediatrics for postgraduate exams

EXAMINATION OF CEREBELLAR SYSTEM

Dysarthria
'Hello, what's your name?' Chat to patient to assess speech

Nystagmus
'Look straight ahead at me' – are the eyes steady?
'Follow my finger with your eyes, keeping your head still'

Dysdiadochokinesis
Show the child that you want him/her to tap with the other, alternately tapping
the palm and the back of the hand

Dysmetria
The child will overshoot the target when asked to point to a target

Intention tremor
'Reach out and touch my finger' – the child's hand is steady at rest but develops a
tremor of increasing amplitude as it approaches its target

Ataxic gait
Ask the child to walk to the end of the ward and back – broad-based gait with
arms stretched out sideways for balance. Difficulty turning corners

Romberg's sign
'Stand with your feet together, close your eyes' – positive if the child becomes
unsteady, due to loss of proprioception (rare in children)

EXAMINATION OF CHILD IN A WHEELCHAIR

INSPECTION
Overall posture, use of wedges for support (hypotonia)
Head size, hydocephalus +/– shunt (spina bifida)
Face – dysmorphic features, myopathy
Shake hands – feel for tone, grip, power and release of grip
Urinary catheter bag (spina bifida)
Splints, supports, calipers (cerebral palsy)

PALPATE
Feel scalp for a shunt/reservoir

DO NOT EXAMINE IN CHAIR
Explain to the examiner you would like to examine the patient on the bed. The
examiner may ask you to examine the upper limbs and arms only
Try to determine the site of paresis:
— head
— cord
— peripheral nerve
— muscular disease

The developmental examination

8

Examiners in both the membership examination and the DCH are encouraged to examine all candidates on their developmental assessment of children. This can be the hardest part of the clinical to do well in and is the most difficult to prepare for. There are a few points about the developmental examination, which you must remember.

- It is an assessment of the acquisition of *learned* skills, which reflect the child's genetic potential and environment.
- Development follows an orderly progress in a *cephalic to caudal direction* (there is little point in being able to walk if you cannot hold your head up and look around) and also requires the loss of the early primitive reflexes (you cannot develop finger–thumb apposition while you still have an active grasp reflex).
- Be opportunistic.
- Present your findings as you go along.
- There are five periods of development, which are part of routine child surveillance:
  — newborn
  — supine (6–8 weeks)
  — sitting (6–9 months)
  — mobile toddler (18–24 months)
  — communicating child (3–4 years).
- There are four fields to assess:
  — *gross motor:* development of locomotion
  — *vision and fine manipulation:* development of hand–eye coordination
  — *hearing and speech:* development of language
  — *personal and social:* integration of acquired abilities to reflect general understanding of the environment.
  It is very important to present the case by referring in a logical fashion to each of these four fields in turn.
- Is development normal or delayed? There is a sequence of development within each field, but the development in one field does not necessarily run parallel with that in another, known as *dissociation* (see Fig. 8.1)

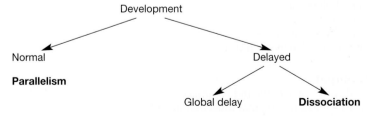

Fig. 8.1 Assessment of development.

Development follows an orderly sequence within each field although the rate of acquisition of abilities is very variable. The significance of delayed development within each field is also variable, with some fields of development being more important than others. Gross motor development is not as important as manipulative development, while the child's alertness, interest in surroundings and concentration are the most important factors in the assessment of mental agility. The ages at which normal children sit and walk can be very variable, with some normal children not walking until 2 years of age. On the other hand, some mentally retarded children may learn to sit and walk at the usual age.

Developmental assessment requires a knowledge of the essential milestones, and failure to acquire them may be considered suspicious. We recommend that you familiarize yourself with the Denver developmental assessment test which describes the different developmental abilities for each age and gives the variation within the normal range. If a child fails to achieve certain milestones within the 90% confidence intervals shown in the chart, appropriate referrals should then be initiated. A guide to assist you with developmental assessment of the child in the exam is given in Table 8.1. This reflects skills which are acquired by 50–75% of children by the ages shown and is not intended to reflect the 'action times' by which stage all children should have acquired these skills; therefore, failure to acquire these skills by the ages shown does not necessarily reflect delayed development.

PRIMITIVE REFLEXES

These appear from birth (Moro, palmar and plantar grasp, stepping) and are then lost as development progresses; persistence beyond these age limits reflects failure of the CNS to mature (Ch. 7, p. 157).

CAUSES OF DELAYED DEVELOPMENT

DELAYED MOTOR DEVELOPMENT

Familial

Environmental
- Emotional deprivation
- Lack of opportunity to practise
- Malnutrition.

Central
- Immaturity – isolated delay
- Variant of normal – bottom-shuffler
- Global mental retardation
- Control movement
  — cerebellar ataxia
  — cerebral palsy
- Organization – apraxia
- Hypotonia – Down's syndrome.

Motor output
- Spinal cord – spasticity and weakness
- Nerves – weakness (spinal muscular atrophy)
- Muscles – weakness (muscular dystrophies)

Table 8.1 Hearing testing (see also Fig. 8.2)

Age	Tests	Procedure
Neonate	Auditory response cradle	Detects behavioural responses to sound
	Auditory brain stem evoked potentials	Measures electrical activity in the brain in relation to sound
6–18 months	Distraction testing	Requires two examiners and parent: one examiner engages the child's attention, while the other presents sound from behind the child. The child sits on the parent's knee and turns the head in response to sound. Test sound is presented at 35 dB and at different frequencies, e.g. 'ooh, ooh' for low tone, and 'ss, ss' for high tone
18–30 months	Cooperative testing	Simple instructions are given by the tester in a quiet voice with the lips covered
24–30 months	Performance test	The child's ability to perform a test is checked (e.g. place a brick in the box – 'conditioning'). The test sound is then reduced and visual clues are avoided
2–4 years	Speech discrimination test	The child identifies objects or pictures. Monosyllabic words whose sounds may be easily confused, e.g. house and cow, man and lamb, are commonly employed. The best is the McCormack toy discrimination test, which uses objects normally within the child's vocabulary
>4 years	Pure tone audiometry	Must be carried out in a quiet environment with acoustic cups placed over the child's ears to cut out background noise. This will test the child's ability to hear sound across the main speech frequencies (500 Hz–4 kHz).
Any age	Oto-acoustic emissions	Measures sound reflected from the normally functioning cochlea
	Tympanometry	Tests for middle ear pathology, in particular 'glue ear'. A sound is passed into the ear and the amount of sound reflected back is measured. The pressure in the external auditory canal is varied and compliance of the tympanic membrane is tested by measuring the reflected sounds at different pressures. In glue ear, reflected sound is reduced, giving a flat curve

- Myopathies
- Structural – mechanical (talipes, CDH).

Special senses
- Interfere with perception of environment – visual impairment.

General disorders
- Hypotonia
  — hypothyroidism
  — chronic hypoxia
- Connective tissue disorders.

DELAYED SPEECH OR ABNORMAL LANGUAGE DEVELOPMENT

Familial

Environmental
- Emotional deprivation
- Paucity of spoken language in the home.

Special senses
- Hearing impairment.

Central
- Global learning difficulties
- Autism
- Cerebral palsy
- Dysphasia.

Twinning 'own language'
Always check that English is the child's first language. The 'delayed' child may be fluent in Urdu.

DELAYED SPHINCTER CONTROL

Familial

Learning difficulties

Environmental
- Mismanagement of toilet training.

Physical
- Meningomyelocele
- Uterocele
- Ectopic ureter (female)
- Urethral valves (male).

HEARING AND LANGUAGE

Hearing loss can be sensorineural (perceptive) or conductive (Fig. 8.2). Early detection of deafness is important to avoid impaired speech, language and learning, and behavioural difficulties.

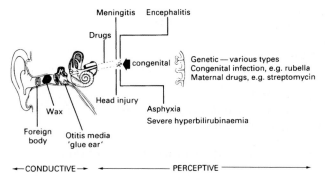

Fig. 8.2 Causes of deafness. (From Polnay L, Hull D (eds) 1993 Community Paediatrics, 2nd edn. Churchill Livingstone, Edinburgh, with permission.)

Children at risk of deafness are those with the following:

- history of meningitis or encephalitis
- cleft palate
- history of recurrent otitis media
- significantly delayed or unclear speech
- cerebral palsy
- parental suspicion of deafness.

HEARING LOSS (Fig. 8.2)

Sensorineural
Incidence is 3/1000.

Hereditary (50%)
- Usher's syndrome (AR) – retinitis pigmentosa also leads to visual loss later
- Pendred's syndrome (AR) – goitrous hypothyroidism
- Jervell–Lange–Nielson syndrome (AR) – long QT syndrome may lead to sudden death
- Wardenburg's syndrome (AD)
  — white forelock of hair
  — heterochromia irides
- Stickler syndrome (AD) – severe myopia
- Pierre–Robin anomaly.

Congenital
- CHARGE syndrome
- Congenital infection – rubella, CMV

Perinatal
- Prematurity
- Birth asphyxia
- Ototoxic drugs (during pregnancy or in neonatal period), e.g. aminoglycosides
- Hyperbilirubinaemia
- Cerebral palsy (particularly athetoid).

Acquired
● Meningitis/encephalitis
● Mumps
● Head injury.

Conductive
Incidence is 5–10/100.
● Down's syndrome – middle ear abnormalities
● Treacher Collins' syndrome
● Goldenhar's syndrome
● Secretory otitis media – especially if cleft palate or Down's
● Wax (rarely leads to deafness).

MANAGEMENT OF CHILD WITH SENSORINEURAL DEAFNESS

You may be asked in the exam: 'Can this child hear?' We recommend the following approach, although formal assessment of the child should be undertaken by a specialist team and you should be able to describe the appropriate tests for each age group (Fig. 8.3).

Enquire of the examiner whether you are allowed to ask the parent. If not, use the following:
● *infant*
— startle response: blink
— head turning to loud handclap or rattle
● *older child*
— performance testing (Table 8.1)
— speech discrimination testing (Table 8.1)
— if the child knows numbers (>4 years old) whisper numbers in one ear and ask him/her to repeat them.

Hearing aids
These will not restore hearing to normal, as high tones are hard to amplify. Hearing aids can be fitted from a few months of age and fitting and follow-up should be performed by the specialist team.

Cochlear implants
Cochlear implants may be indicated for profoundly deaf children but are currently indicated primarily for children who have lost their hearing after learning to speak (e.g. post-meningitis). Cochlear implants can be intra- or extra-cochlear. Electrodes are inserted into or onto the surface of the cochlea

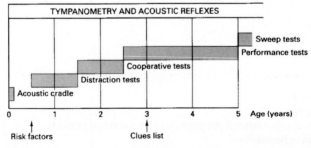

Fig. 8.3 Screening tests for hearing. (From Polnay L, Hull D (eds) 1993 Community Paediatrics, 2nd edn. Churchill Livingstone, Edinburgh, with permission.)

and attached to a receiver inserted under the skin behind the pinna. The child wears a microphone which transmits sound to the receiver. For selected children with maximal support from a specialist centre, this is proving to be an exciting new development.

MANAGEMENT OF CONDUCTIVE HEARING LOSS

The natural history of serous otitis media is for it to resolve spontaneously with time. Medical management is usually unrewarding. Surgical management with myringotomy and adenoidectomy, with or without grommets, is commonly used for short-term improvement in young children and can be of benefit to their language development.

Communication methods

Total communication, a combination of speech, signs, lip reading, gesture and body language, is commonly taught to children with profound hearing losses. Manual methods, e.g. British Sign Language, have their strong advocates but their major disadvantage is that they do not facilitate integration of the child into the hearing world.

VISION

Severe visual handicap has a prevalence of 1 in 2500 children in the UK. Children with a visual acuity of 3/60 in the better eye are registered blind and children with a corrected visual acuity in the better eye of 4/60–6/24 are registered partially sighted.

Factors which may be associated with a visual defect

General
- Behaviour problems or educational failure
- Family history of blindness, squint or amblyopia.

Congenital
- Congenital rubella infection
- Craniostenosis.

Perinatal
- Prematurity
- Severe pre-eclampsia: risk of myopia
- Hydrocephalus
- Cerebral palsy
- Ophthalmia neonatorum.

You may be asked in the exam: 'Can this child see?' We suggest a simple approach for the exam setting, although you must be able to describe the appropriate formal assessments that would be necessary if any abnormalities were detected (Table 8.2).

General inspection of the eye before vision testing   Look for:

- nystagmus (roving)
- lens opacity
- absence of red reflex
- ptosis (may be bilateral)
- strabismus
- abnormal pupillary responses.

Table 8.2 Testing visual acuity

Age	Test
4 weeks	Fix on mother's face
	Catford drum
	Preferential looking test – preference for patterned objects as opposed to plain
	Visual evoked potentials
6 weeks	Fix and follow object 90 cm away through 90° (but not beyond midline): use a 4 cm red ball or pen torch. Turn the light on and off intermittently
	Optokinetic nystagmus – demonstrated on looking at a moving, striped target
3 months	Follows object 90 cm away through 180° while lying supine
10 months	Identifies small objects, e.g. raisin, in the palm of the hand and can pick up with pincer grip. Test with each eye covered. A 1-year-old can pick up individual 'hundreds and thousands'
2–3 years	Miniature toys – using a chair, doll, car, plane, spoon, knife and fork, the majority of children can identify all seven toys. Familiarize the child with all the toys and then, at a distance of 3 m, ask: 'What's this?' If the child cannot speak intelligibly, give him/her a duplicate set of toys, to indicate the answer. Test both eyes and then each eye in turn
3 years	Stycar matching letters: the first letters a child learns are V, O, X, H and T, and later A, U, I and C. Once the child is familiar with the procedure, he/she matches letters in their set with letters held up by the examiner at distance of 3 m. The size of the letters decreases and visual acuity can be assessed. Test both eyes and each eye in turn. Near vision is tested in the same way using a near vision chart at about 46 cm
>5 years	Snellen charts – most children are able to read the chart sitting in front of a mirror at 3 m (i.e. 6 m)
	Ishihara plates – used in boys to test for colour vision from about 10 years old

If the child is able to communicate   Cover one eye and ask them to count fingers.

● If this is successful you can older ask an older child to read text appropriate for his/her age.
● If the child is unable to count fingers because of an inability to see them, ask whether he/she can see your hand waving.
● If the child is unable to see your hand waving, ask him/her to distinguish between light and dark.

If a child is unable to communicate   Test for:

● ability to fix and follow with red ball
● ability to reach for object
● menace reflex.

Causes of blindness

In decreasing order of prevalence.

- Optic atrophy
- Congenital cataracts
- Choroidoretinal degeneration
- Malformation of eye
- Retrolental fibroplasia
- Myopia
- Albinism
- Retinoblastoma
- Uveitis.

Normal visual development (Fig. 8.4)

Visual acuity
- Neonate – 6/200
- 3 months – 6/60
- (5 months – adult colour vision)
- 12 months – 6/18
- 3 years – 6/6.

Visual screening The purpose of visual screening is to detect severe visual handicap, which may be treatable, e.g. cataract, and to detect moderate visual problems, which may cause problems with reading, and to prevent amblyopia.

SQUINT

Definition A squint *(strabismus)* is present if one eye is not directed towards the object under scrutiny. A squint may be:

- paralytic (incomitant) or *concomitant* (non-paralytic)
- divergent or *convergent*
- latent or *manifest*
- *unilateral* or bilateral
- *permanent* or intermittent
- *horizontal* or vertical.

The more common variants are shown in italic type.

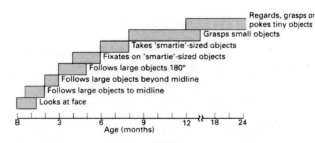

Fig. 8.4 Development of visually directed behaviour. (From Polnay L, Hull D (eds) 1993 Community Paediatrics, 2nd edn. Churchill Livingstone, Edinburgh, with permission.)

- 50% of children have a family history of squint or refractive error; therefore siblings should also be assessed.
- Squints per se are not inherited, but the factors causing the squint may be inherited.

Aetiology

Paralytic   The angle subtended by the eyes varies with the direction of the eye. It is rare, though common in children with cerebral palsy and mental retardation.

   Paresis of extraocular muscles   Cranial nerve palsies (normal control of eye movements are shown in Fig. 8.5):
- III – divergent squint
- IV and VI – convergent squint.

A VIth nerve palsy may be associated with raised intracranial pressure. When squint is of rapid onset, an underlying space-occupying lesion must be excluded.
   Weakness of extraocular muscles
- Myogenic lesions – usually congenital conditions associated with musculofacial abnormalities
- Duane's retraction syndrome (fibrosis of external rectus muscle)
- Superior oblique tendon sheath syndrome (Brown's syndrome).

Concomitant (non-paralytic)   The angle of deviation remains unchanged whatever the direction of gaze.
   Type
- Convergent or divergent
- Hypertropic (eye turns upwards) or hypotropic (eye turns downwards)
- Horizontal or vertical (occasionally both)
- Permanent or intermittent (occasionally present only on fixation for certain distances or in certain direction of gaze).
   Causes
- Refractive error – hypermetropia is the commonest leading to overconvergence and a convergent squint
- Failure to develop binocular vision

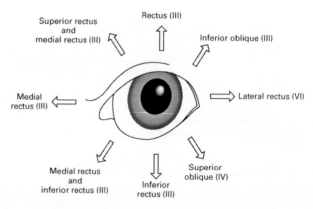

Fig. 8.5 Normal control of eye movements.

● Eye disease
    — cataracts
    — retinoblastoma
    — corneal scar
    — retinopathy of prematurity.

Pseudo-squint   Visual axes are correctly aligned but child appears to have a squint. It is common in young children but tends to disappear with facial development. It is confirmed by a negative cover test.
    Causes
● Marked epicanthic folds (bilateral or unilateral)
● Small or large interpupillary distance
● Broad nasal bridge
● Facial asymmetry.

Heterophoria (latent squint)
● Due to extraocular muscle imbalance creating a potential deviation
● Causes are similar to those for manifest squint
● Generally less problematic than manifest squint
● Generally only requires correction of a refractive error
● Can deteriorate to true squint during illness or change in refractive error.
    Causes
● Esophoria – tendency for eyes to *turn in* due to either *convergence excess* on near vision or *divergence weakness* on distance vision
● Exophoria – tendency for eyes to *turn out* due to either *divergence excess* or *convergence weakness*
● Hyperphoria – tendency for eyes to *turn upwards*
● Hypophoria – tendency for eyes to *turn downwards*.

Assessment of the child with a squint
1. Remove spectacles.
2. Check visual acuity of each eye independently.
3. Observe the position of the child's eyes. If a paralytic squint is present, the angle subtended by the eyes will vary with the direction of gaze.
4. Look at the corneal reflections of a bright light held 30 cm in front of the eyes. The position of the reflections on the eyes should be symmetrical.

Cover tests   There are two types, which may be used to reveal a squint.
    Cover/uncover test   One eye is covered and the other is observed. If the uncovered eye moves to fix on the object there is a squint, which is present all the time – a *manifest squint* (Fig. 8.6). The test should be carried out by covering each eye in turn.
    Alternate cover test   If the cover/uncover test is normal, which indicates that no manifest squint is present, the alternate cover test should be used. The occluder is moved to and fro between the eyes and if the eye which has been uncovered moves, a *latent squint* is present (Fig. 8.6).

Careful examination of the optic fundus   The purpose of screening for squints is to detect refractive problems, diagnose underlying eye disease, and prevent amblyopia (the suppression of vision in a structurally and functionally normal eye).

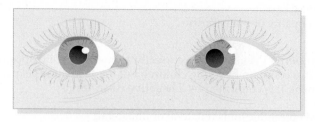

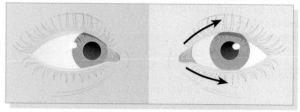

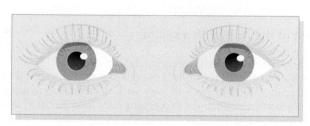

a

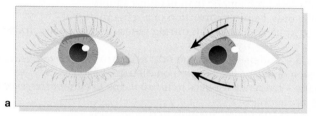

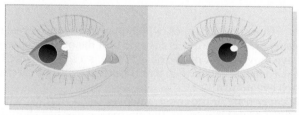

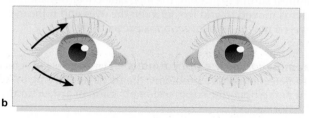

b

ABNORMALITIES OF REFRACTION

Emmetropia is the condition in which no refractive error is present and parallel rays are brought to a point focus on the macula when the eye is at rest.

Hypermetropia (long sight)

This is the commonest refractive error and is due to the eyeball being slightly shorter than normal so that rays of light are focused behind the retina. Near vision will be impaired and is treated with glasses using convex lenses.

Myopia (short sight)

The eye is too large and therefore parallel rays of light are brought into focus in front of the retina. The myopic child will have difficulty with distant vision. This usually develops between 7 and 14 years of age. There is usually a positive family history and the condition is treated with glasses using concave lenses.

Astigmatism

The curvature of the cornea and lens is different in the horizontal and vertical planes and parallel rays of light are not brought to a point focus when the eyes attempt to accommodate. Even with simple spherical glasses, the images will always be blurred for both near and far vision and thus the child must wear lenses incorporating a cylinder to correct the astigmatism.

SERIOUS VISUAL IMPAIRMENT IN CHILDREN

Each year in the UK more than 450 children under 15 years of age are registered blind or partially sighted. The importance of recognizing visually handicapped children is threefold.

● Early treatment may prevent visual disability or reduce its severity.
● Genetic counselling, medical and social support can be provided as required.
● Some of the causes of blindness are associated with systemic disease.

◀ **Fig. 8.6**   The cover/uncover test for squint
The cover test is based on the fact that if there is no squint and normal binocular vision, both eyes maintain steady fixation on a distant object and there will be no deviation when either eye is covered. When there is a manifest or latent squint deviation of the eye will be seen on occlusion of one or other eye. (a) In manifest convergent squint, the squinting eye is turned in and the non-squinting eye maintains fixation. If the squinting eye is occluded there will be no variation in the angle of the squint, but when the non-squinting eye ('fixing eye') is occluded, it converges and the squinting eye takes up fixation. When the occluder is removed the original position is resumed. (b) In latent squint, both eyes will fix a distant object but when one eye is covered it deviates. When the cover is removed, the eye with the latent squint resumes fixation. The other eye does not shift or lose fixation while the opposite eye is being covered or uncovered.

Causes of visual impairment in children can be divided as follows:

- cataract
- optic nerve pathology (e.g. optic nerve glioma)
- retinal pathology (e.g. retinitis pigmentosa)
- trauma to any part of the eye
- albinism
- glaucoma
- nystagmus
- delayed visual maturation
- cherry red macular degeneration of Tay–Sachs disease.

Visual loss before the age of 2 years is usually accompanied by:

- 'roving' eye movements
- persistent hand regard
- lack of blink to menace
- nystagmus.

Cataract

Bilateral opacification of the lens accounts for up to 30% of visually handicapped babies. The diagnosis is suggested by absence of the normal pupillary red reflex (ophthalmoscope held 30 cm away with +4 convex lens).

The *three main causes* of congenital cataract are:

- familial
- secondary to prenatal infections (rubella, syphilis but not toxoplasmosis)
- associated with prematurity.

Other conditions associated with cataract are:

- Down's syndrome
- children on continuous corticosteroid treatment
- trauma to the eye
- diabetes mellitus
- myotonic dystrophy
- hypoparathyroidism and any cause of hypocalcaemia
- Lowe's syndrome
- secondary to lens dislocation (Marfan's, homocystinuria)
- secondary to aniridia
- galactokinase deficiency
- galactosaemia.

Early removal of cataract with optical correction can offer an excellent visual prognosis.

Optical nerve pathology

Optic nerve pathology blinds as many children as cataract but is less amenable to treatment. Most causes of optic atrophy are inherited. The optic disc of normal babies is pale and can be difficult to distinguish from optic atrophy.

Causes

- May be associated with cerebral palsy
- Septo-optic dysplasia (absence of septum pellucidum and associated with hypopituitarism)

- Intracranial tumours and hydrocephalus
- Leber's hereditary optic atrophy – rarely presents in young children.

Retinal pathology

Retinopathy of prematurity (ROP)
- Predominant cause of retinal pathology
- May be associated with cataracts
- More common in premature babies weighing <1500 g
- All high-risk babies should be screened at 34 weeks post-conceptual age.

Retinoblastoma
- Must be excluded in any child presenting to hospital with a visual defect
- Incidence of 1 in 18 000 live births
- Present initially with a squint alone in about 33% of cases
- Cardinal clinical sign of loss of the red reflex
- 20–30% bilateral
- 40% inherited – affected parent, unaffected carrier parent or new mutation
- Autosomal dominant inheritance – gene mutation 13q14.

Toxoplasmosis
- Typical 'clock-face' macular scar (the phakoma of tuberous sclerosis is usually at the optic disc).

Retinitis pigmentosa
- Leber's amaurosis (AD)
- Refsum's syndrome
- Abetalipoproteinaemia
- Laurence–Moon–Biedl syndrome
- Mucopolysaccharidoses.

Choroidoretinitis
- Congenital
- Toxoplasmosis
- CMV
- Syphilis
- Toxocariasis
- Tuberculosis
- Sarcoidosis.

Histoplasmosis

Corneal clouding
- Hurler's syndrome
- Congential glaucoma
- Keratitis
- Post-traumatic
- Post-infectious (HSV, HZV)
- Cystinosis
- Wilson's disease
- Hypercholesterolaemia
- Hypercalcaemia
- Fabry's disease.

Glaucoma

Congenital glaucoma (buphthalmos) presents with:

- globe enlargement
- clouding of the cornea
- photophobia.

Associated conditions include:

- Sturge–Weber syndrome
- aniridia (absence of iris bilaterally).

Nystagmus (see also Ch. 7)

Visual loss before the age of 2 years is usually accompanied by nystagmus; however, nystagmus due to unstable ocular fixation will lead to a reduction in measured visual acuity.

MANAGEMENT OF VISUAL IMPAIRMENT

- Assess for associated disabling conditions, e.g. hearing loss.
- Provide genetic counselling where indicated.
- Provide emotional support for child and family.
- Recommend the use of low vision aids and games to encourage the child's use of any residual vision.
- Assess educational placement to optimize the child's developmental progress.

PRINCIPLES OF HEALTH SURVEILLANCE

- Child health surveillance should be carried out in partnership with parents.
- It should be a positive experience with opportunities to exchange information and provide sensible guidance on behaviour, nutrition, accident prevention and immunization of young children.
- The health visitor is the major health professional engaged in child health surveillance of pre-school children, whereas the school nurse is the key person for children of school age.

DEVELOPMENTAL SCREENING

A child's development is assessed at various time points during the first 5 years of life and there are a number of milestones that should be met at each stage. A guide for the milestones easily tested for in the exam setting are outlined in Table 8.3, but we recommend that you familiarize yourself with formal developmental screening tests such as the Denver developmental test. This outlines the normal variation for acquisition of skills, beyond which point development may be delayed and the appropriate referral should be made. Table 8.4 outlines the important questions to ask the parents and the particular features to check for during the examination in order to assess the child's development.

PARENT-HELD CHILD HEALTH RECORDS

There are a number of advantages to parent-held child health records, which have been used in parts of the UK since the late 1970s. The main advantages are:

- there is good evidence that parents do not lose these records
- a record is available wherever the child is seen
- a record is available as the family relocates
- confidentiality rests with parents
- parents can record their own observations.

The developmental examination

Table 8.3 A guide to developmental assessment of the child in the exam setting

	Gross motor	Vision/fine motor	Hearing/speech	Personal/social
6 weeks	Symmetrical limb movements Ventral – head in line with body briefly Supine – fencing posture Automatic stepping and walking	Fixes and follows to 90° Turns to light Grasp reflex	Cries/coos Startles to noise	Smiles
3 months	Moves limbs vigorously No head lag Back – lumbar curvature only Prone – lifts upper chest up	Fixes and follows to 180° Plays with own hands Holds rattles placed in hand	Quietens to mother's voice Turns to sound	Laughs and squeals
6 months	Sits without support Lifts chest up on extended arms Grasps feet Rolls front to back Downward parachute	Palmar grasp Transfers objects Shakes rattle Mouths objects	Turns to quiet sound Says vowels and syllables	Laughs and screams Not shy
9 months	Tripod sits – rights self if pushed and can reach for toy steadily Rolls back to front Pulls to standing Stands holding on Forward parachute (7 months)	Reaches for small objects Rolls balls Points with index finger Early pincer grip Looks for fallen objects Releases toys	Distraction hearing test Says 'mama', 'dada', non-specifically	Chews biscuit Stranger anxiety Plays 'peek-a-boo' Understands 'no' and 'bye-bye'
12 months	Cruises around furniture Walks if held, may take a few steps unsupported	Neat pincer grip Casting objects Bangs cubes together	Knows name Understands simple commands Says few words	Drinks from cup and uses spoon Finger-feeds Waves 'bye-bye' Finds hidden object

The developmental examination

Table 8.3 *(continued)*

	Gross motor	Vision/fine motor	Hearing/speech	Personal/social
15 months	Broad-based gait Kneels Pushes wheeled toy	Sees small objects Tower of 2 bricks To and fro scribble	2–6 words Communicates wishes and obeys commands	Uses cup and spoon
18 months	Steady purposeful walk Runs, squats Walks carrying toy Pushes/pulls Creeps downstairs	Circular scribble Points to pictures in book Turns pages of book Hand preference	6–20 words	Points to named body parts Feeds independently Domestic mimickry Symbolic plays alone Takes off socks and shoes
2 years	Kicks ball Walks up and down stairs holding on	Tower of 6 bricks Copies vertical line	2–3 word sentences Uses pivotal grammar Uses question words	Feeds with fork and spoon Begins toilet training Temper tantrums
3 years	Walks up stairs 1 foot per step, down with 2 Walks on tip-toes Throws ball Pedals tricycle	Tower of 9 bricks Builds train and bridge with bricks if shown Copies circle	Gives first and last name Knows sex Recognizes colours Pure tone audiometry	Washes hands and brushes teeth Eats with fork and spoon (+/–knife) Make-believe play Likes hearing and telling stories
4 years	Walks up and down stairs 1 foot per step Hops	Builds steps of bricks Copies cross Draws man	Counts to 10 or more	Able to undress
5 years	Skips Catches ball Runs on toes	Copies triangle	Asks 'how' and 'when' questions Uses grammatical speech	Uses knife and fork Able to put on clothes and to do large buttons

Table 8.4 Developmental screening

	Neonate	6 weeks	8–10 months	3–4 years	5 years
History	Pregnancy and delivery Any parental concerns	Birth details Illness to date Age of onset of: — smiling — vocalization Response to sound Sucking and swallowing difficulties Risk factors for DDH – FH, breech, caesarean section, talipes, torticollis, plagiocephaly Any parental concerns	Birth details As for 6 weeks plus: Age of onset of: — holding rattle — turning to sound — reaching out and getting object — sitting — chewing — crawling — stand holding on (10 months) — waves 'bye-bye' (10 months) Any words (10 months) Any parental concerns	Birth details As for 8–10 months plus: Age of onset of: — walking alone — joining words together — extent of vocabulary — speech understandable to strangers — toilet trained Ability to dress and feed himself Diet: iron deficiency peaks at 3 years Immunization history Any parental concerns	Any parental concerns: — hearing — vision — speech — behaviour — general health — school Immunization history Any important life events
Examination	Measure and record weight, length, OFC Observe alertness Dysmorphic features? Inspect — eyes: red reflex — mouth for cleft palate CVS/RS/GI/spine/feet Genitalia: — testes descended — hypospadias — cliteromegaly Hips: — developmental disclocation — Barlow and Ortolani tests	Measure and record weight, length, OFC Dysmorphic features Fontanelle Eyes – red reflex, squint, nystagmus CVS/RS/GI/genitalia Spine/hips Hold in ventral position Place prone Pull to sitting from supine Test weight bearing Test reflexes if tone or posture abnormal Test primitive reflexes (not essential)	Measure and record weight, length, OFC Dysmorphic features Fontanelle Eyes – red reflex, squint, nystagmus CVS/RS/GI/genitalia Pull to sitting; sitting ability Observe grasp of raisin – test each eye Finger–thumb apposition Test weight bearing Assess tone and reflexes if indicated Distraction hearing test Hips – assess for DDH by hip abduction	Measure and record weight, height, OFC Dysmorphic features General physical exam Hip abduction Gait Standing on one leg/hop Manipulation of small objects Drawing a man Speech Test hearing and vision	Plot height and weight Visual acuity – Snellen chart Test hearing Examination – hair/skin/teeth/posture Interaction with parents

Skin

9

The dermatological cases you are most likely to see in the exam are those not uncommonly found on acute paediatric wards (e.g. eczema, drug rash, erythema multiforme, purpura), which may be incidental to the reason for admission, or chronic cases which can be arranged easily in advance of the examination day (e.g. psoriasis, dermatitis herpetiformis). Alternatively, if you are taking the exam in a large centre or children's hospital in which there is a specific paediatric dermatology ward or infectious diseases unit, you may see some very rare rashes indeed! Many of the conditions mentioned in this chapter are extremely rare in general paediatric practice but you will be expected to suggest a list of differentials for a number of common dermatological presentations, such as generalized, maculopapular rash, an itchy rash and a circumscribed patch of decreased pigmentation.

Examination of the 'skin'
Ensure the prepubertal child is completely undressed. Inspect the following:

- hair
- nails
- skin
- mucous membranes
- teeth.

Congenital variants are discussed in Chapter 12 and the skin abnormalities associated with the neurophakomatoses are discussed in Chapters 7 and 11.

HAIR

ABSENCE

Localized
- Alopecia areata – look for exclamation mark hairs at the edge of the patch; the cause is unknown
- Trichillomania (hair pulling); short hair roots are usually present
- Ringworm
- Short occipital hair may occur in a child with motor delay who is left supine for much of the time. Patchy alopecia also occurs in deprivation.

Generalized
- Alopecia totalis may develop from areata
- Cytotoxic therapy

- Following cranial irradiation
- Following 'total' shave for neurosurgery
- Ectodermal dysplasia – look for associated dental hypoplasia and absent nails in this rare sex-linked recessive disorder.

ABNORMALITIES OF THE HAIR

- Coarse facial hair – chronic phenytoin therapy
- White forelock – Waardenburg's syndrome
- Bushy eyebrows (synophrys) – Cornelia de Lange syndrome, mucopolysaccharidoses
- Kinky hair – Menkes' syndrome
- Hirsuteness
  — Asian infants
  — drug induced:
    — phenytoin
    — diazoxide
    — ciclosporin A.

NAILS

- Pitted nails in psoriasis
- Beau's lines – a transverse ridge corresponding to arrested nail growth during a severe illness
- Paronychia is common in newborn infants
- Fungal infection may cause separation of the nail from the bed (onycholysis)
- Splinter haemorrhages under the nail are seen in bacterial endocarditis
- Deformed nails in epidermolysis bullosa
- Absent nails in ectodermal dysplasia
- Koilonychia (spoon-shaped nails) is a sign of chronic severe iron deficiency anaemia and is rarely seen nowadays
- Leuconychia (diffusely white nails) is a result of chronic hypoalbuminaemia in nephrotic syndrome and liver disease
- White spots on the nails are a normal variant.

SKIN

DESCRIBING A SKIN LESION

Dermatologists make the subject more difficult than it need be by couching their terminology in Latin phrases and using confusing classifications. For the paediatrician, the best approach is to describe exactly what you see in plain English.

The skin is the only organ visible to the outside world and is the interface with both our physical and our social environment. Try to empathize with the child, anticipating how the stigma of an abnormality of the skin may affect him/her.

Define a skin abnormality as follows:

Single or multiple

Site   Centripetal or centrifugal

Size
- Uniform or varied
- 'Morbilliform' – macules similar to those in measles
- 'Rubelliform' – macules similar to those in rubella.

Colour
- May vary between lesions
- May be strikingly different from the surrounding skin, e.g haemangioma
- Alternatively, there may be more subtle variations in the shade of flesh colour:
  — vitiligo: depigmented patches
  — lentigines: brown spots, as in the acronymous leopard syndrome
  — hypopigmentation and hyperpigmentation (see below)
  — café-au-lait spots and axillary freckling (see Chs 7 and 11).

Shape   Common usages are:

- discoid
- nummular – coin-shaped
- confluent
- multiforme – 'of many shapes' and is not confined to the target lesions of erythema multiforme
- target lesions
- annulare
- umbilicated – with a central depression, as in the lesions of molluscum contagiosum, but not on a stalk as many candidates think.

Surface   Many rashes are itchy but very few are painful or infectious.
Palpation of a skin lesion is all too often forgotten. *Common terms* are:

- macule – flush with the skin
- papule – raised above the surrounding skin
- marginatum – edge is raised, as in erythema marginatum
- lichenified – thickened
- ichthyotic – dry and scaling.

HYPOPIGMENTATION

May be localized or generalized.

Local
- Previous inflammation, e.g. herpes zoster
- Burn or scar
- Vitiligo – usually bilateral and symmetrical, associated with alopecia areata and autoimmune disease
- Shagreen patches – tuberous sclerosis
- Pityriasis versicolor – fungal infection
- Pityriasis alba – associated with atopic dermatitis, usually affects the face and sometimes the upper arms.

General
- Albinism (AR) – pink pupils, blue irides, white hair
- Phenylketonuria (AR) – blonde hair and blue eyes

- Hypopituitarism – short stature and micropenis
- Chediak–Higashi syndrome (AR) – blonde hair, blue to brown eyes, neutrophil phagocyte defect, thrombocytopenia, increased risk of malignancy and decreased IQ
- Hermansky–Pudlak syndrome – blonde hair, blue-grey eyes platelet disorder.

HYPERPIGMENTATION

May be localized or generalized.

Local
- Previous inflammation
- Pigmented naevus or melanoma
- Café-au-lait spots
  — significant: > six, each >1.5 cm
  — neurofibromatosis (type I)
  — Albright's syndrome (polyostotic fibrous dysplasia and sexual precocity in females)
- Peutz–Jeghers syndrome (AD) – pigmented spots in or around the mouth often associated with gastrointestinal bleeding
- Chronic phenytoin therapy
  — gum hypertrophy
  — coarse, hirsute facies
- Leopard syndrome – lentigines, ECG abnormalities, ocular defects, pulmonary stenosis, abnormal genitalia, retarded growth, deafness.

General
- Racial or suntan
- Haemosiderosis (e.g. multiple transfusions for thalassaemia)
- Addison's disease
- Primary biliary cirrhosis.

ITCHY RASHES

May indicate:

- eczema
- psoriasis
- contact dermatitis
- dermatitis herpetiformis – associated with coeliac disease
- fungal infections – tinea or 'ringworm' (a confusing misnomer since it includes tinea capitis, tinea corporis and tinea pedis).

The following, although common, are unlikely to be seen in an exam:

- urticaria/allergic reactions
- insect bites
- chickenpox
- scabies
- pityriasis rosea (herald patch)
- pediculosis capitis – the nits, or eggs, of lice cause itching of the scalp.

Visual clues suggesting that a skin condition is itchy are:

- excoriation
- the wearing of mitts
- Koebner phenomenon.

KOEBNER PHENOMENON

Itching or trauma to previously unaffected skin results in fresh lesions:

- psoriasis
- lichen planus.

Infective skin lesions such as warts and impetigo can be spread by scratching, but this is not the true Koebner phenomenon.

PALMS AND SOLES

Lesions which may affect the palms or soles are:

- warts/verrucae – human papilloma virus. Common in children >4 years old; usually resolve spontaneously within 3 years
- erythema multiforme
  — inflammatory condition of skin and mucous membranes with many causes, e.g. herpes simplex, *Mycoplasma*, drugs
  — minor or major forms occur
  — Stevens–Johnson syndrome (severe bullous form)
- hand, foot and mouth disease – Coxsackie A
- desquamation
  — Kawasaki's disease
  — post-streptococcal infection
  — following friction (common blister, e.g. on the heel from new shoes)
  — separation of the epidermis: Nikolsky's sign, seen in staphylococcal scalded skin syndrome in the newborn, also known as Lyell's or Ritter's disease, but unlikely to be seen in the exam
- pustular psoriasis
- pompholyx – a bullous form of eczema
- malignant melanoma.

Lesions which 'never' affect palms or soles are:

- benign naevus (common 'mole')
- sebaceous cyst
- lipoma.

BLISTERS, VESICLES AND BULLAE

These are all fluid-filled lesions.

- Vesicle – <0.5 cm
- Bulla – >0.5 cm by convention
- Blister – the result of friction or a burn
- Pustule – a vesicle which contains pus
- Boil – a collection of pus in the skin but not preceded by a clear vesicle.

The *differential diagnosis* of a skin condition *depends on the age* of the child:

Neonate
- Bullous impetigo – staphylococcal skin infection (rarer scalded skin syndrome is due to a staphylococcal exotoxin)
- Herpes simplex
- Epidermolysis bullosa – autosomal recessive forms are severe; autosomal dominant forms are milder. Look for old scars and nail deformities
- Incontinentia pigmenti – X-linked dominant, only seen in girls, as fatal in boys. Look for old scars, hyperpigmented whorls and dental abnormalities.

Child
- Insect bites
- Chickenpox
- Herpes zoster
- Herpes simplex
- Dermatitis herpetiformis – usually confined to buttocks or genitalia
- Erythema multiforme – rarely seen in exams.

HAEMORRHAGES IN THE SKIN

Haemorrhages into the skin *do not blanche* with pressure, which helps distinguish these from telangiectasia and erythema, which are due to dilated skin blood vessels.

Haemorrhages are defined by size.

- Petechiae – <1 mm in diameter
- Purpuric spots – 2–10 mm in diameter
  - *palpable*: vasculitic
    - Henoch–Schönlein purpura
    - meningococcaemia
  - *non-palpable*: thrombocytopenia
- Ecchymoses – larger bruises
- Haematoma – haemorrhage large enough to produce a tender elevation of the skin.

Aetiological classification of skin haemorrhage
Virchow's triad specifies that there are three components of the coagulation system (vascular endothelium, platelets and clotting factors) and that an abnormality of any of these may result in haemorrhage.

Vascular abnormalities
- Henoch–Schönlein purpura
- Meningococcal septicaemia
- Increased fragility
  - chronic steroid effect
  - Ehlers–Danlos syndrome
  - vitamin C deficiency (scurvy).

Thrombocytopenia
Increased consumption of platelets
- Idiopathic thrombocytopenia purpura
- Iso-immune thrombocytopenic purpura – rare cause of thrombocytopenia in the newborn, analogous to iso-immune haemolysis of red cells

- Haemolytic uraemic syndrome
- Disseminated intravascular coagulation
- Hypersplenism
- Wiskott–Aldrich syndrome – thrombocytopenia, eczema and increased susceptibility to infection; affects boys only
- Kasabach–Merritt syndrome – large cavernous haemangiomas in skin or abdominal viscera.

  Decreased production of platelets
- Leukaemia
- Cytotoxic drugs
- Aplastic anaemia due to certain drugs, familial (Fanconi's anaemia) or idiopathic
- Thrombocytopenia with absent radius – TAR syndrome.

  Defective platelet function
- von Willebrand's disease – qualitative platelet defect and factor VIII deficiency; an autosomal dominant condition with variable expression.

Abnormal clotting

- Haemophilia A – X-linked recessive factor VIII deficiency
- Haemophilia B (Christmas disease) – X-linked recessive factor IX deficiency
- von Willebrand's disease (see above)
- Haemorrhagic disease of the newborn – vitamin K deficiency
- Chronic liver disease – vitamin K deficiency
- Too much warfarin – antagonizes vitamin K.

COMMON LONG CASES

ECZEMA

First, a word of clarification about terminology. Eczema and dermatitis are synonymous, describing a red itchy rash, which may be dry or moist and sometimes raised and thickened. However, dermatitis is used more often to describe the skin abnormality in adults in whom it is often a reaction to a specific environmental trigger. The term atopic eczema is used for the condition, commonest in early childhood and often resolving by puberty, in which the aetiology of the skin disorder remains unclear but is part of a wider constitutional atopy. Although specific allergens may give positive skin tests, exposure to these seems to bear little relevance to clinical fluctuations in the disease.

HISTORY

When did the rash first appear?

- Usually within first 2 years of life
- 2 years may carry a worse prognosis
- <3 months is unusual for truly atopic eczema (seborrhoeic dermatitis is a more likely diagnosis)
- Affects 5–10% of children
- Often preceded by a monilial or ammoniacal nappy rash or by seborrhoeic dermatitis.

Where did the rash first appear?   Infantile eczema usually affects the cheeks and limb flexures. If the initial lesions were confined to extensor surfaces, and particularly if the first attack was not until school age, consider psoriasis.

Was the infant breast- or bottle-fed?   There is some evidence that avoidance of cow's milk protein early in life protects against later atopy and therefore the incidence is lower in children who were breast-fed. However, the relationship between cow's milk protein and the risk of atopy is not dose-dependent and breast-feeding must be completely exclusive until the age of 3 months to confer this advantage. Some would argue that the breast-feeding mother should also be on a diet free of cow's milk protein.

Does the child have a special diet?   Dietary elimination may be considered in children who fail to respond to topical therapy. The main allergens are cow's milk, egg, soy and wheat. Dietary elimination should be carried out under the supervision of a dietician. Tolerance to offending foods usually develops as the child gets older.

Does the child also suffer from asthma or allergic rhinitis, seasonal ('hay fever') or otherwise?

Is there a family history of eczema, asthma or hay fever?   First-degree relatives have, or have had, some form of atopy in over 50% of cases.

How has the eczema affected the child's self-image and has it resulted in teasing at school?   Severe eczema is very trying for the parents as well as the child, so ask about sleepless nights, frequency of hospital visits and admissions, and fears about the cosmetic outlook.

EXAMINATION

Patches of eczema are usually:

- red
- itchy
- raised
- excoriated
- of different sizes
- symmetrical.

Distribution of atopic eczema (predominant areas)
- Infant – face
- Young child – extensor surfaces
- Older child – flexor surfaces.

What to look for
- Eczema may be dry or weeping.
- In severe cases the rash may be very widespread and accompanied by generalized lymphadenopathy.
- Look for local (thin skin or striae) and systemic side-effects of steroid therapy, and for evidence of bacterial superinfection (yellow scabs or pustules).
- Always examine the respiratory system carefully for any signs of chronic or active asthma.

Always plot the child's height and weight on an appropriate centile chart as severe eczema can adversely affect growth, not least because of severe and inappropriate dietary restrictions.

MANAGEMENT

Ask specifically about the following measures.

Avoiding irritants
- Avoiding woollens and synthetic fibres next to the skin
- Avoiding 'biological' washing powders for clothes
- Measures to reduce scratching:
  — trimming fingernails and toenails
  — cotton mitts
  — bandaging of affected limbs
  — calamine lotion or coal tar ointment (especially for lichenified lesions)
  — night sedation.

Emollients
- Hydrous ointment and aqueous cream, applied frequently to prevent the skin drying
- Emulsifying ointment instead of soap
- Reducing the frequency of baths and adding oil to the bath water.

Topical steroids
- This is the most effective treatment for eczema but must be used with care.
- In mild to moderate eczema the least potent topical steroids should be used and restricted to periods of 1–2 weeks, in conjunction with regular use of emollients.
- Severe eczema on the limbs or body – application of a potent or moderately potent corticosteroid for the first 1–2 weeks, followed by a weaker preparation as the condition improves.
- The order of increasing potency is:
  — hydrocortisone
  — clobetasone butyrate (Eumovate)
  — betamethasone (Betnovate)
  — clobetasol proprionate (Dermovate).

Antibiotics or antibacterial agents
- The use of topical or systemic antibiotics for secondary infection
- The antiviral agent aciclovir is given for eczema herpeticum.

Occlusive bandages
- These are helpful when itching and lichenification are a problem.
- Wet dressings of potassium permanganate are applied if there is weeping eczema and potassium permanganate baths can be taken if the area is large.
- Coal tar has potent anti-inflammatory and anti-scaling properties and can be used to treat chronic atopic eczema, and zinc paste and coal tar bandages can be applied to the limbs.
- Ichthammol has a milder action than coal tar and is usually used in chronic lichenified forms of eczema. It can be applied to the limb flexures as zinc paste and ichthammol bandages.

Antihistamines

Itch can be suppressed with H_1 histamine antagonists given at night.

Dietary elimination

- This can be considered in those not responding to topical treatment.
- The main food allergens are cow's milk, eggs, soy and wheat, although any food may be implicated.
- A response is usually achieved after 3–4 weeks of dietary elimination.
- A dietician should be involved to ensure that the diet is nutritionally adequate.
- Tolerance to certain foods is often seen as the child gets older.

Oral immunosuppressants

Ciclosporin may be used for severe resistant atopic eczema only in the context of specialist care in a hospital.

Immunization

Atopic eczema is *not a contraindication* to any of the standard immunizations given to children in the UK, including the measles vaccine.

COMMON SHORT CASES

- Purpura
- Café-au-lait patches
- Adenoma sebaceum
- Incontinentia pigmenti
- Sturge–Weber syndome

PURPURA

Purpura is easily recognized and is a common physical sign in the short cases. Table 9.1 presents an easily remembered scheme for differentiating the aetiology. This is not meant to be a comprehensive list of the causes of purpura but these are the commonest causes to be met in the exam. Always remember to exam the whole 'skin' system and exam for lymphadenopathy and hepatosplenomegaly.

More detail on the short cases can be found in Chapter 1 and in *Paediatric Short Cases for Postgraduate Examinations* by A Thomson, H Wallace and T Stephenson (Churchill Livingstone, Edinburgh, 2003).

Table 9.1 Purpura

	Normal platelets	Low platelets
'Nice'	Henoch–Schönlein purpura Whooping cough Vitamin C deficiency	Idiopathic thrombocytopenic purpura
'Nasty'	Non-accidental injury Meningococcal septicaemia (purpura is classically necrotic) Clotting disorders	Acute lymphoblastic leukaemia Haemolytic uraemic syndrome Disseminated intravascular coagulation Hypersplenism

The musculoskeletal system

10

Clinically, the correct sequence for assessing joint pathology is 'look, feel, move, measure, X-ray'. Whilst the benefit of radiographs is not usually available at postgraduate exams (although they are sometimes used during short cases in the DCH), this approach is still valid.

LOOK

General inspection
- Thriving?
- Any bandages, splints, plaster of Paris or traction?
- In a wheelchair?

Spinal deformities
- Kyphoscoliosis.

Limb deformities
- Amelia is absence of a limb
- Hemiamelia is absence of the distal half of a limb
- Phocomelia is when the hand or foot is attached directly to the trunk
- Contractures
- Joint swellings.

Skin
- Erythema
- Trophic skin changes.

Muscles
- Muscle wasting (disuse atrophy).

FEEL

Always ask whether any part of the limb is painful and what exacerbates the pain. Although technically this is part of the history, it is an essential enquiry to make before touching the limb. Pain in a joint may cause spasm of adjacent muscles, although this is not usually detectable clinically, and the joint is usually held in midflexion as this position places minimum tension on the joint capsule. Pain in the knee may be referred from the hip joint and pain in the hip/thigh from the lower back.

PALPATION OF THE JOINT

Starting from an area of normal skin some distance away from the affected joint for comparison, feel for:

- skin temperature – use back of hand
- tenderness – in response to palpation, as opposed to pain which may be present all the time. Anticipate the possibility of tenderness by starting with very gentle palpation and *watch the child's expression*; a heavy-handed approach looks inexperienced and unsympathetic.
- enlargement – the most common detectable site is the knee joint:
  — effusion (more likely with an acute arthropathy)
  — synovial thickening (more likely with a chronic arthropathy)
  — bony enlargement
  — all three of the above.

TESTING FOR AN EFFUSION

Use the palm of the left hand to massage the fluid down from the synovial space above the patella and, maintaining pressure with the left hand, press with the thumb of the right hand over the medial aspect of the knee. The tense, fluid-filled swelling should be palpable 'bimanually' and this technique is much more sensitive, and a lot less painful, than a positive 'patellar tap'.

MOVE

ACTIVE BEFORE PASSIVE MOVEMENTS

It is impossible to memorize the normal range of movements at every joint, especially since it varies with age and sex, but much can be learned by comparing left and right limbs or comparing an older child to yourself.

- Elbow – 140º
- Wrist – 180º
- Knee – 140º.

Establish whether joint movement is limited by:

- pain
- contracture
- muscle weakness
- neurological spasticity.

EXAMINATION OF THE JOINTS

It is important to have a well-rehearsed system for examining all the joints of the body, to enable quick and efficient examination of the child in the long case, or adaptation for the short case. The most straightforward and easily memorable way is to start with the head and work down.

- Always ask if the child is sore anywhere.
- Begin with the child sitting on the edge of the bed.
- The degree of movement is measured from the neutral position, i.e. imagine the child is lying supine, with the head in the midline and the feet at a 90° angle to the bed.
- Demonstrate the movements to the child to help him/her understand your commands.

Neck (Fig. 10.1)
- Flexion – 'Put your chin on your chest'
- Extension – 'Look up at the ceiling'
- Lateral rotation – 'Look over your shoulder'
- Lateral flexion – 'Put your ear on your shoulder'.

Temporomandibular joint (Fig. 10.2)
'Open your mouth as wide as possible and see if you can insert your second, third and fourth fingers into it.'
  If the joint is affected, crepitus can be felt as you palpate over the joint.

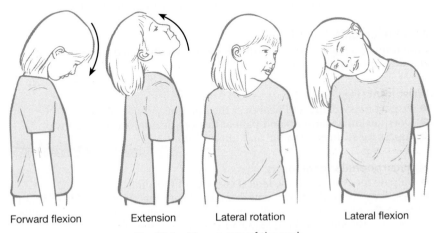

Forward flexion   Extension   Lateral rotation   Lateral flexion

Fig. 10.1   Movements of the neck.

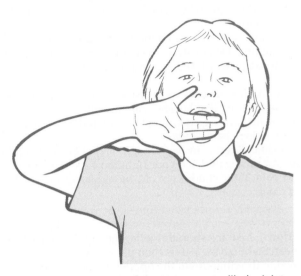

Fig. 10.2   Assessment of the temporomandibular joint.

Shoulder joint (Fig. 10.3)
- The joint itself is too deep to see swelling or feel heat.
- All movements are tested *passively*.
- Need to stabilize the shoulder girdle. Place one hand firmly upon the patient's shoulder and use your other hand to move the arm in order to test flexion, extension, abduction, superior and inferior rotation, when the arm is abducted to 90°.

Elbow joint (Fig. 10.4)
- Look for swelling and feel for heat (comparing with other arm)
- Synovial swelling, if present, can be palpated below the lateral epicondyle as a boggy area; if not hot – chronic synovitis
- Flexion – 140°
- Extension – 180°; if unable to fully extend, the patient has a fixed flexion deformity and is measured as the number of degrees short of 180°.

Radioulnar joint (Fig. 10.5)
Pronation and supination with the elbow flexed and fixed to prevent shoulder movement.

Wrist joint (Fig. 10.6)
- Inspect for swelling and heat over the dorsum.
- Dorsiflexion (extension) and palmar flexion (flexion) are 90° each way.
- Assess for stiffness at radial and ulnar joints.

Metacarpophalangeal joints
- Palpate for swelling at the lateral surfaces of the joints.
- Best way to assess movement – 'make a fist'; the child should be able to bend the fingers to 90° at all joints. It is also easier to observe for swelling between the joints when making a fist.
- If there is distal interphalangeal joint swelling, look at the nails for pitting.

Spine (Fig. 10.7)
- With the child still sitting, so that the pelvis is splinted, ask him/her to rotate the torso through 90° to assess rotation of the spine. It is easier to demonstrate this to the child.
- Flexion, extension, rotation and lateral flexion can be done at the end once the child is standing. Demonstrate the manoeuvres to the child first.
  — flexion: 'Bend forward and try to touch your toes keeping your legs straight'
  — extension: 'Arch your back as far backwards as you can.' Stand behind the child to reassure that he/she will not fall!
  — rotation: 'Keep your legs pointing forward and try to turn the top part of your body to look behind you.'
  — lateral flexion: 'Keep your legs straight and slide your right hand down the side of your leg to touch your right foot.' Do the same with the other side and point if the child is not old enough to know which are the right and left sides.

Hip joint
Lie the child down. Like the shoulder joint, the hip is too deep to assess for swelling or heat. Stabilize the pelvis then passively test abduction, adduction, flexion (holding down the opposite leg) and internal and external rotation (with the hip and knee at 90°).

a

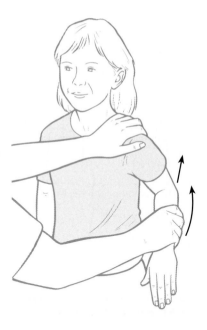

Stabilize the shoulder joint and passively extend the arm backwards behind the patient

b

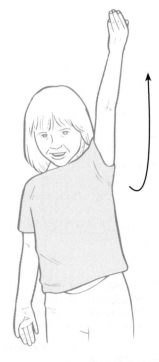

Bring the arm forward and fully flex the arm above the shoulder joint

c

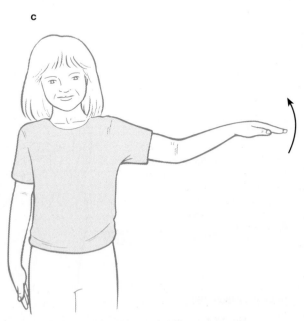

Fig. 10.3 Assessment of the shoulder joint. (a) Extension; (b) flexion; (c) abduction.

d

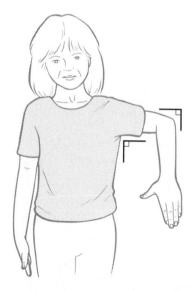

Abduct arm to 90° at shoulder joint
then rotate shoulder superiorly by
elevating forearm to 90°

Rotate shoulder inferiorly by rotating
forearm at elbow to 90° to the
horizontal

Fig. 10.3 *contd*   (d) Superior and inferior rotation.

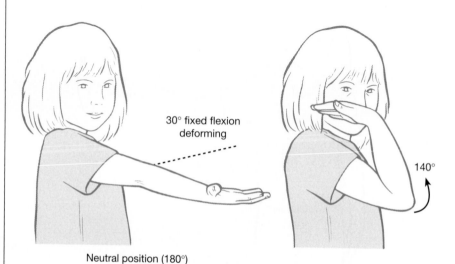

30° fixed flexion
deforming

140°

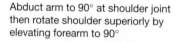

Neutral position (180°)

Fig. 10.4   Assessment of the elbow joint.

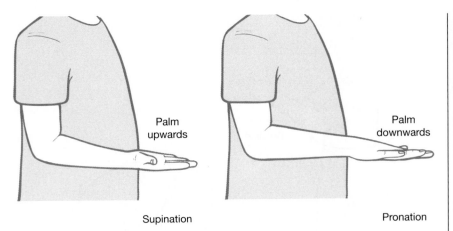

Supination

Pronation

Fig. 10.5 Assessment of the radioulnar joint.

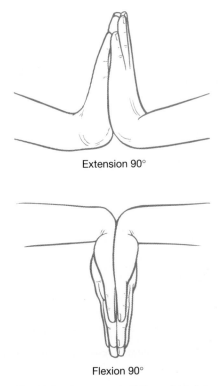

Extension 90°

Flexion 90°

Fig. 10.6 Assessment of the wrist joint.

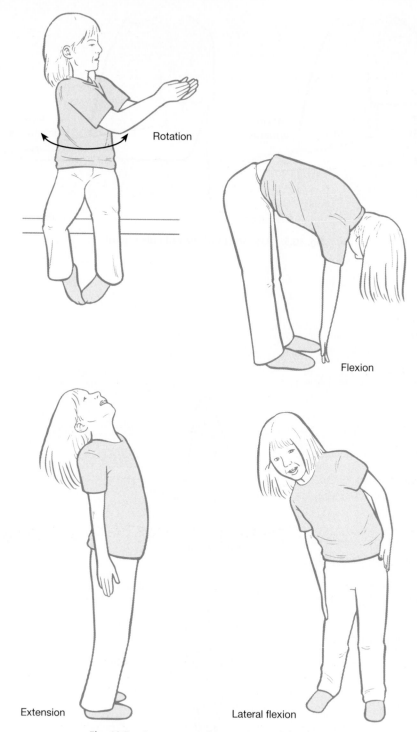

Rotation

Flexion

Extension

Lateral flexion

Fig. 10.7   Assessment of movements of the spine.

Knee joint

This is the most frequently affected joint and the most commonly examined in exams.

Look for:
- effusions – the absence of indentations just above the patella
- deformities – valgus and varus.

Feel for:
- heat
- effusions (patellar tap).

Move
- Extension – 'Push down on my hand' – the child will be able to squash your hand if there is normal extension.
- Flexion – 'Bend your knee and pull your heel up towards your bottom'.

Ligament stability is not usually tested in the exam situation.

Ankle joint (three joints)

Look for swelling *from behind* – absence of indentations on either side of Achilles tendon.

Tibiotalar joint
- Dorsiflexion – 'Pull your toes up to your head'
- Plantarflexion – 'Point your toes into the bed'.

Subtalar joint
- Inversion and eversion – test passively by stabilizing the lower leg and rocking the heel back and forward.

Midtarsal joints   Medial and lateral movements of the forefoot: test passively.

Metatarsal joints

Look for dactylitis.

MEASURE

LIMB CIRCUMFERENCE

Limb circumference is measured from a set point above (e.g. 10 cm) and below (e.g. 5 cm) the tibial tuberosity to look for muscle wasting.

LIMB LENGTH

There may be scoliosis due to pelvic tilt but to assess leg length properly, the child must lie on a flat surface and leg length is measured from the anterior superior iliac spine to the medial malleolus with a tape measure (Fig. 10.8).

- True leg length – anterior superior iliac spine to medial malleolus
- Apparent leg length – pubic symphysis to medial malleolus.

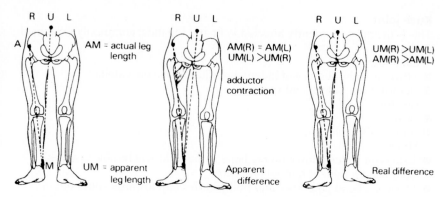

Fig. 10.8 Real and apparent differences in leg length. (Reproduced with permission from Milner A D, Hull D (eds) 1984 Hospital Paediatrics. Churchill Livingstone, Edinburgh.)

Causes of a *true difference* in leg length are:

● undetected congenital dislocation of the hip
● previous trauma or bony surgery
● increased limb growth due to arthritis of the knee
● severe hemiparesis – this can also cause an apparent difference in leg length because adductor spasm causes pelvic tilt
● osteogenesis imperfecta – look for blue sclerae and hyperextensible joints
● Ollier's disease
● polyostotic fibrous dysplasia (café-au-lait patches and sexual precocity in girls)
● hemihypertrophy usually results in a difference in girth but may also alter length. Associations are:
— idiopathic
— Wilms' tumour (look for associated aniridia)
— neurofibromatosis
— arteriovenous malformation
— diastometamyelia.

DEFORMITIES

SCOLIOSIS

● Inspect from behind with the child standing.
● Describe the side of the scoliosis as the side to which the spine is convex.
● The shoulder on the convex side is elevated.
● Curvature of the spine:
— flexion: kyphosis
— extension: lordosis
— lateral: scoliosis
● Inspect from behind with the child standing. Ask the child: 'Can you touch your toes?'
● If scoliosis *disappears* = postural (80%)
— idiopathic (adolescent female)
— unilateral muscle spasm secondary to pain
— unequal leg length.

- If *fixed* = structural (20%). There is a gibbus, or hump, due to increased convexity of the underlying ribs (secondary to rotation of the vertebrae), on the side of the convexity:
  — idiopathic
  — Marfan's syndrome
  — neurofibromatosis
  — muscular dystrophy.

Scoliosis is *associated with*:

- Sprengel's shoulder – one scapula is fixed in a high position due to failure to descend during fetal development. There is limited abduction of the shoulder and there may be hypoplasia of the shoulder girdle muscles. There may also be a cervical rib (and therefore brachial plexus compression)
- Klippel–Feil syndrome – the fundamental defect is fusion of the cervical spine. This results in short neck, low hairline and webbing of the skin of the neck (differential diagnosis is Turner's syndrome). There is restricted neck movement and sometimes torticollis. There may also be cervical spina bifida and thoracic hemivertebrae (and hence root or cord compression).

KNEE DEFORMITIES

Bow legs (genu varum)
- Due to bowing of the tibiae
- Common in children under 3 years
- Seldom needs treatment
- Orthoses and surgical correction may be required in Blount disease (infantile tibia vara):
  — marked bow legs due to beaking of the proximal medial tibial epiphysis on X-ray
  — uncommon disease seen in Afro-Carribean children.

Knock-knees (genu valgum)
- The feet are wide apart when standing with the knees together
- Common between 2 and 7 years of age
- Generally self-resolving.

FOOT DEFORMITIES

Flat feet (pes planus)

Benign flat feet   Toddlers generally have flat feet when learning to walk due to flatness of the medial longitudinal arch and the presence of a fat pad which later disappears.

Failure of arch to develop   This is demonstrated by absence of an arch when standing on tip-toes. It occurs in:

- collagen disorders
  — Ehlers–Danlos syndrome
  — Marfan's syndrome
- cerebral palsy.

Surgery is only required in symptomatic adolescents.

High-arched feet (pes cavus)
- Spina bifida
- Diastometamyelia – weakness and sensory impairment in the legs, possibly bladder problems and unequal lower limb growth due to spinal cord tethering
- Friedreich's ataxia – cerebellar ataxia, pyramidal tract signs, dorsal column sensory loss and scoliosis
- Charcot–Marie–Tooth disease – peroneal muscular atrophy and absent leg reflexes.

In-toeing
There are three main causes.

- Metatarsus varus – an adduction deformity of a highly mobile forefoot
- Medial tibial torsion – the lower end of the tibia is less laterally rotated than normal
- Persistent anteversion of the femoral neck – the femoral neck is twisted more forward than normal.

Out-toeing
- Uncommon
- May occur in 6- to 12-month-old infants
- If bilateral, it is due to rotation of the hips and resolves spontaneously.

Toe-walking
- Common in 1- to 3-year-olds
- May persist due to:
  — habit
  — cerebral palsy
  — tight Achilles tendon with no neurological deficit
- Duchenne's muscular dystrophy should be excluded in older boys.

Talipes equinovarus (club foot)
- Affects 1 in 1000 births
- Twice as common in males
- 50% are bilateral
- Foot is inverted and supinated and forefoot abducted, with heel rotated inwards in plantarflexion
- Multifactorial inheritance
- Secondary to oligohydramnios during pregnancy
- Part of malformation syndrome
- Spina bifida cystica
- Peroneal muscular atrophy (Charcot–Marie–Tooth syndrome: 'champagne bottle' muscle wasting in the legs and dorsal column sensory loss)
- May be associated with congenital dislocation of the hip
- Treatment is started promptly with stretching and strapping or serial plaster casts. Corrective surgery is required if severe.

Talipes calcaneovalgus
- Foot is dorsiflexed and everted
- A consequence of intrauterine moulding
- Self-correcting.

Minor anomalies

- Syndactyly of second/third toes is common and often familial
- Overlapping of the third, fourth or fifth toes is common.

NEONATAL HIP EXAMINATION

In the United Kingdom, every newborn infant undergoes a screening examination for congenital dislocation of the hips (CDH). Despite this, children continue to present at an older age with undiagnosed CDH, but what remains unclear is whether the CDH was missed during the screening exam or whether the hips became dislocated later, i.e. not every case may be strictly 'congenital'. It remains for large trials to be carried out to demonstrate whether ultrasound examination in the newborn period can reduce the incidence of these late presentations. True dislocation is rare (except in spina bifida) but unstable or 'clicky' hip occurs in approximately 1% of neonates.

In the newborn, the classic signs of dislocation, such as asymmetrical skin folds, limited abduction and an apparently shortened femur (Galeazzo's sign), are usually absent; these signs are secondary and do not usually develop until the age of 6 weeks. CDH in the immediate newborn period is diagnosed by using two 'provocation manoeuvres' to demonstrate that the femoral head can be dislocated and then lifted back into the acetabulum.

BARLOW AND ORTOLANI MANOEUVRES

Lie the infant supine on a flat hard surface and remove the nappy. Start with the infant's knees together and the hips and knees held flexed at 90° with your thumbs on the medial condyles of each femur and the tips of the middle fingers on the greater trochanters of each femur. Now attempt to push the hips posteriorly (down into the bed); if you feel a 'click', the head of the femur has dislocated and *Barlow's sign* is positive.

Now, keeping your grip unchanged, lift the femoral heads forward with the middle fingers while you abduct the thighs with your thumbs. If you feel a definite 'clunk' (the femoral head returning to the acetabulum) the dislocation is reducible and *Ortolani's sign* is positive. These signs remain positive in CDH up to 6–8 weeks of age, but thereafter negative provocation tests do not exclude CDH, as the hip may be permanently and irreducibly dislocated. The secondary signs discussed above then become much more significant.

CONGENITAL DISLOCATION OF THE HIP (CDH)

- Six times more common in girls than in boys
- Affects left hip more commonly than right hip
- Positive family history in 20%
- Associated with:
  - breech presentation
  - neuromuscular disorders: neural tube defect
  - torticollis
  - talipes calcaneovalgus.

- Child with a limp
- Juvenile idiopathic arthritis

CHILD WITH A LIMP

An acute limp is usually the result of pain, especially joint pain, occurring anywhere from the toe to the spine. *Commonest causes* are:

- verruca or other source of pain in the foot
- local trauma, including occult fracture
- irritable hip (usually boys)
- reactive viral arthritis.

Less common causes are:

- juvenile chronic arthritis
- bacterial arthritis
- osteomyelitis
- Osgood–Schlatter disease (usually boys)
- chondromalacia patellae (usually girls)
- Perthes' disease (usually boys)
- slipped femoral epiphysis
- malignancy, particularly acute lymphoblastic leukaemia, or neuroblastoma
- Henoch–Schönlein purpura with arthropathy
- inguinal hernia.

Juvenile chronic arthritis and Perthes' disease are probably the most common causes encountered in the MRCP exam.

A chronic limp is more likely to be seen in the postgraduate examinations than an acute limp and is more likely to be the result of a deformity or weakness rather than pain. Club foot is one of the commonest congenital abnormalities, usually talipes equinovarus (ankle inverted and plantar flexed).

- Inspection – deformities, scars, rashes, joint swelling, etc.
- Ask the child to walk
- Are the leg lengths equal?
- Site of problem – need to examine hip, knee and ankle, but first ask about the site of pain.

JUVENILE IDIOPATHIC ARTHRITIS

Juvenile idiopathic arthritis (JIA) refers to a group of conditions in which there is, by definition, chronic arthritis that persists for a minimum of 3 months (6 weeks in USA) in one or more joints, before the age of 16 years, and after active exclusion of other causes. It is estimated to affect 1 in 1000–5000 children.

HISTORY

- How did the child first present?
- Joint swelling, painful joints, limp, systemic symptoms
- Which joints are involved?

- Treatment (see below) including joint injections
- Ask about the child's growth and development and specifically enquire about growth hormone therapy
- Impact of the condition on the child and family life?
- How much school has the child missed?
- Are there any limitations on the child's physical activities?

EXAMINATION

Ask if the child has any pain anywhere and then proceed to examine all the joints as described previously, including measurement of limb length.
Look specifically for associated features.

- Rheumatoid nodules – on pressure points, particularly elbows
- Skin/nails – psoriatic arthropathy
- Hepatosplenomegaly – in acute systemic presentation but unlikely in exam
- Vasculitis – uncommon and often late, nailfold lesions and ulceration
- Anterior uveitis – inform the examiner that you would like the child to be tested for this using a slit lamp
- Flexion contractures of the joints
- Growth failure – make sure you plot the child's height and weight on a growth chart appropriate for age and sex
- Injection sites – if on growth hormone
- Pubertal assessment – often puberty will be delayed.

MANAGEMENT

A multidisciplinary team approach is required to ensure that the treatment is optimal and the family and patient are provided with all the education and psychological support they require. This should include the following:

- physiotherapy
- occupational therapy
- chiropody
- orthotics
- psychologist
- GP/specialist paediatrician/nurse/teacher
- drugs
- surgery.

Drugs

NSAIDs   Pain control and suppression of inflammation
Steroids
- Oral/i.v. – for severe uveitis, systemic disease, immobility, severe polyarthritis, pericarditis
- Intra-articular.
Immunosuppressants   Requires careful monitoring of side-effects.
- Methotrexate – very effective in seronegative polyarthritis, psoriasis, but only for a few years until the disease burns out
- Ciclosporin – can be added in if the patient is not responding to methotrexate
- Sulfasalazine – useful in enthesitis.

Drugs not used in JIA
- Salicylates
- Penicillamine
- Gold
- Antimalarials.

POINTS FOR DISCUSSION

Classification
Have an understanding of the classification of juvenile chronic arthritis and how the categories differ clinically. The classification is determined by mode of onset in the first 6 months and often depends on the number of joints involved, systemic features, the presence of rheumatoid factor and enthesitis (inflammation of the insertion of tendons into bone).

- Systemic (9%)
- Polyarticular – rheumatoid factor negative (16%)
- Polyarticular – rheumatoid factor positive (3%)
- Oligoarticular – persistent (≤4 joints) (49%)
- Oligoarticular – extended (after 6 months involves >4 joints) (8%)
- Enthesitis-related arthritis (usually B27-associated) (7%)
- Juvenile psoriatic arthritis (8%)
- Unclassified (1%).

Differential diagnosis
Despite the unknown aetiology of the majority of disorders described, differentiation is important because of varying complications, management and prognosis. When the diagnosis is unknown it is important to take an accurate history, including age of onset, sex, race, preceding illnesses, recent travel, duration of symptoms and family history. The differential diagnosis for JIA is:

- infection
- neoplasia
- blood dyscrasias
- mechanical anomalies, including injury
- biochemical abnormalities
- genetic and/or congenital abnormalities
- connective tissue disorders.

New therapies
- Role of immunomodulators, e.g. anti-TNFα antibodies, and immunoglobulins
- Potential role of autologous stem cell transplantation.

Long-term side-effects of drugs
Be able to discuss the unwanted long-term side-effects of steroids, NSAIDs and imunossuppressants.

COMMON SHORT CASES

- Monoarthropathy
- Psoriatic arthropathy
- Arthropathy secondary to haemophilia

MONOARTHROPATHY

Infection is the commonest cause of an acute monoarthropathy, but in any child with monoarthropathy or polyarthropathy, acute or chronic, show the examiners that you are aware of possible systemic aetiologies:

- *Juvenile idiopathic arthritis* – offer to examine the eyes for iridocyclitis and look for hepatosplenomegaly and lymphadenopathy
- *Haemarthrosis* – look for bruising or petechiae which suggest haemophilia. Ask about trauma
- *Henoch–Schönlein purpura* – look at the legs and buttocks for palpable purpura (vasculitis)
- *Rheumatic fever* – feel for rheumatic nodules, listen for a cardiac murmur, and ask about any recent sore throat
- Typical scaly rash on exterior surfaces and nail pitting of psoriasis.

The short cases are discussed in more detail in *Paediatric Short Cases for Postgraduate Examinations* by A Thomson, H Wallace and T Stephenson (Churchill Livingstone, Edinburgh, 2003).

SUMMARY OF MUSCULOSKELETAL EXAMINATION

JOINT EXAMINATION
Do not forget to examine gait
Always ask – is it sore anywhere?

LOOK, FEEL, MOVE
As with the other systems observation is an essential part of the examination.
Look for: thriving, splints, bandages, plaster casts, traction, wheelchair, limb deformities, etc.
Always ask whether there is pain in the limbs or joints
Start with the head and work down. Begin with the child sitting on the edge of the bed
The degree of movement is measured from the neutral position

Neck
Extension – 'Look up at the ceiling'
Flexion – 'Put your chin on your chest'
Lateral rotation – 'Look over your shoulder'
Lateral flexion – 'Put your ear on your shoulder'
(*Never* ask a child to do a full rotation of the neck)

Temporomandibular joint
'Open your mouth as wide as possible and see if you can insert your second, third and fourth fingers into it'
If the joint is affected crepitus can be felt

Shoulder joint
The joint itself is too deep to see swelling or feel heat. Need to stabilize the shoulder girdle
All movements are tested passively
Flexion, extension, abduction, superior and inferior rotation when abducted to 90°

Elbow joint
Look for swelling and feel for heat (comparing with other arm). Synovial swelling, if present, can be palpated below the lateral epicondyle as a boggy area; if not hot – chronic synovitis. Flexion and extension. Full extension = 180°; if unable to fully extend the patient has a fixed flexion deformity and is measured as the number of degrees short of 180°

Radioulnar joint
Pronation and supination with the elbow flexed and fixed to prevent shoulder movement

Wrist joint
Inspect for swelling and heat over the dorsum
Dorsiflexion (extension) and palmar flexion (flexion) = 90° each way
Assess for stiffness at radial and ulnar joints

Metacarpophalangeal joints
Palpate for swelling at the lateral surfaces of the joints
Best way to assess movement – 'Make a fist'. The child should be able to bend the fingers to 90° at all joints. It is also easier to observe for swelling between the joints when making a fist. If there is distal interphalangeal joint swelling, look at the nails for pitting

Spine
With the child still sitting, so that the pelvis is splinted, ask him/her to rotate the torso through 90° to assess rotation of the spine
Flexion, extension, rotation and lateral flexion can be done at the end once the child is standing

Hip joint
Lie the child down. Like the shoulder joint, the hip is too deep to assess for swelling or heat. Stabilize the pelvis then passively test abduction, adduction, flexion (holding down the opposite leg) and internal and external rotation (with the hip and knee at 90°).

Knee joint
This is the most frequently affected joint and the most commonly examined joint in exams
Look for the absence of indentations at the side of the patella indicating effusion
Look for valgus and varus deformities. Feel for heat and effusions (patellar tap)

● Extension – 'Push down on my hand' – can squash hand if normal extension
● Flexion – 'Bend your knee and pull your heel up towards your bottom'

Ligament stability is not usually tested in the exam situation

Ankle joint (three joints)
Look for swelling from behind – absence of indentations on either side of Achilles tendon
Tibiotalar joint – dorsiflexion and plantarflexion
Subtalar joint – inversion and eversion, stabilize the lower leg and rock the heel back and forward
Midtarsal joints – medial and lateral movements of the foot

Metatarsal joints
Look for dactylitis

Measure
Limb circumference is measured from a set point above and below the tibial tuberosity to look for muscle wasting
Leg lengths are also important, as arthritis of the knee will cause increased growth of that limb which will result in a scoliosis

● True leg length – anterior superior iliac spine to medial malleolus
● Apparent leg length – pubic symphysis to medial malleolus

Common exam syndromes

11

The purpose of this chapter is to focus your attention on groups of associated clinical signs, which constitute paediatric syndromes. There are many common, and some not so common, but characteristic syndromes which candidates for paediatric postgraduate exams are expected to recognize. There is no substitute for wide clinical experience backed by reference to a comprehensive atlas, but an intelligent, logical approach to the dysmorphic child can be practised.

Almost every candidate will encounter a child with a syndrome at some point in the clinical exam. This must be viewed as a chance to score well. If you recognize that a child has Williams syndrome and you have been asked to examine the cardiovascular system, you should be well on your way to a diagnosis.

In this chapter we present a routine for assessing the dysmorphic child and discuss some of the features of some of the more common dysmorphic syndromes which appear in exams, with the aim of sharpening your ability to look for associated clinical signs. This is by no means intended to be a comprehensive list, nor have we included all the clinical features of each syndrome.

THE DYSMORPHIC NEONATE

The question of whether a neonate is dysmorphic or not is a common clinical problem and one that is sometimes asked in the short cases. When faced with a baby who is 'funny-looking', it is important to have a logical clinical approach. Statements such as 'this baby has low-set ears and a degree of hypertelorism' are only acceptable if you can define precisely what you mean, and what measurements you need to make. A summary of the descriptive terms used in dysmorphology is given in Table 11.1.

In response to the question 'Do you think this is a normal looking baby?', we suggest the following systematic approach to inspection, asking yourself the questions detailed.

CRANIUM

- Is there micro-, macro- or hydrocephaly present? (Offer to measure the maximum head circumference.)
- Is the shape normal?
- Is craniosynostosis present?
- Is the occiput flat or prominent?

Table 11.1 Descriptive terms used in dysmorphology

Term	Feature described
Hypertelorism	Increased distance between the eyes
Hypotelorism	Decreased distance between the eyes
Blepharophimosis	Narrowed palpebral fissures
Synophyris	Medial fusion of the eyebrows
Nasal bridge	Upper part of nose between eyes
Alae nasi	Lateral border of nostril
Columella	Medial part or septum of nostril
Philtrum	Vertical folds on upper lip
Pterygium	Webbing, e.g. of the neck = pterygium colli
Syndactyly	Fusion of digits
Pre-axial polydactyly	Extra digit(s) on lateral border of limb
Postaxial polydactyly	Extra digit(s) on medial border of limb
Clinodactyly	Incurving usually of fifth digit
Brachydactyly	Short fingers or toes
Camptodactyly	Bent and contracted digits
Ectrodactyly	Cleft hand or foot
Symphalangism	Fusion of phalanges
Phocomelia	Absence of limb
Rhizomelia	Shortening of proximal segment of limb
Mesomelia	Shortening of middle segment of limb
Acromelia	Shortening of distal segment of limb
Dysplasia	Generalized abnormality of development, e.g. skeletal dysplasia

EYES

● Is there hypo- or hypertelorism? Figure 11.1 illustrates the measurements required to estimate the interpupillary distance from Figure 11.2, after which you can refer to Figure 11.3 to determine if there is an abnormality.

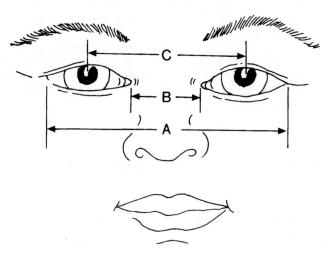

Fig. 11.1 A: outer canthal distance; B: inner canthal distance; C: interpupillary distance – difficult to measure precisely and should therefore be estimated from Figure 11.2 after inner and outer canthal distances have been measured.

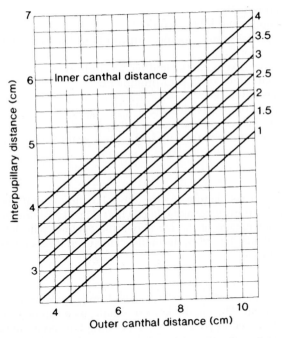

Fig. 11.2 Chart to estimate interpupillary distance from inner and outer canthal distances.

Hypertelorism is seen in:
— idiopathic hypertelorism
— Alpert's syndrome
— Waardenburg's syndrome
— Crouzon's syndrome.

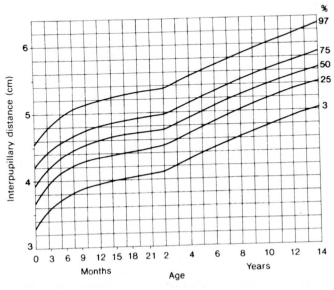

Fig. 11.3 Age-specific norms for interpupillary distance, with key percentiles designated.

- Is there microphthalmus?
- Are medial epicanthic folds present?
- Are the palpebral fissures slanted (upwards in Down's syndrome, downwards in Treacher Collins')?
- Do the eyebrows extend to the midline (synophyrys)?
- Are the orbital ridges shallow or prominent?
- Is there ptosis of the eyelids?
- Are colobomata of the iris present?
- Is there corneal clouding or a lens opacity present?
- Are the sclerae blue (a normal finding up to 1 year of age)?

EARS

- Are the ears low-set? Figure 11.4 describes how to assess if ears are low-set. Referral to the appropriate age-related chart (Fig. 11.5), once you have determined the percentage of the ear above the eyeline, will determine if the child falls outside the 3rd–97th centiles. However, low-set ears alone *do not* make a syndrome.
- Are the ears small?
- Are there preauricular tags?
- Are the ears malformed? The external auricle may be deformed or the meatus narrow or absent. The child's left ear should be examined by holding the auriscope like a pen in your left hand, pointing the speculum (which should be appropriate to the size of the child) forwards, while gently pulling the auricle back with the right hand in order to straighten the external canal. Perforations are more likely in the upper part of the drum. The mother must be shown how to hold the child's head firmly against her chest throughout.

FACE

- Is the face flat, round, broad or triangular?
- Does the nose look normal?

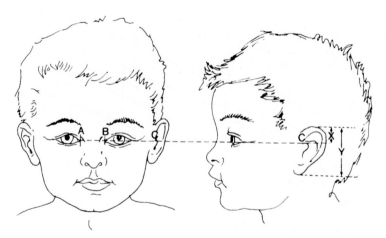

Fig. 11.4 Assessing for low-set ears. A central horizontal line is drawn through the medial canthi (A and B) and extended laterally to point C where it meets the ear. The percentage of ear above the eyeline is calculated from measurement of X and Y.

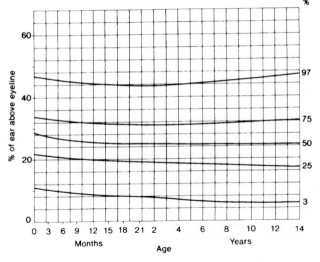

Fig. 11.5   Age-specific norms for percentage of ear above the eyeline.

- Is there a low nasal bridge?
- Is there malar or maxillary hypoplasia?
- Is there micrognathia or prognathia?
- Is the philtrum normal?
  - — long in Cornelia de Lange syndrome
  - — smooth in fetal alcohol syndrome.
- Are the gums ulcerated or hypertrophied (phenytoin)?
- Is there a cleft of the lip or palate present? Is the palate high or arched?
- Are the lips pouting or full? Do the lips show oedema, pallor, cyanosis or ulceration?
- Are the tonsils present and do they look infected?
- Look at the teeth for number, pigmentation and caries.
- Is macroglossia present?
- Are mouth ulcers, thrush or Koplik's spots present?

HANDS AND LIMBS

- Is there a single (simian) crease?
- Are the fingers normal?
  - — brachydactyly
  - — clinodactyly
  - — polydactyly
    - — pre-axial: thumb side
    - — post-axial: little finger side
  - — arachnodactyly
  - — syndactyly.
- Are the thumbs and/or toes broad?
- Is there aplasia or hypoplasia of the radius?

SKIN (see also Ch. 9)

● Is there alopecia or hirsutism?
● Are there abnormalities of pigmentation?
● Is the hair normal?

GENITALIA

● Is there hypospadias, micropenis or cryptorchidism?

During your examination it may become immediately apparent that the neonate has a well recognized syndrome, in which case you should search for additional features of the syndrome and demonstrate them to the examiners. If the dysmorphic features do not add up to a syndrome which you recognize, then it becomes important to list the positive and negative findings along the lines described above, so that you would be able to refer at leisure to a suitable reference book. Below we describe the clinical features of some of the most common syndromes likely to be encountered in the exam, but a more detailed picture of the examination findings associated with these conditions is presented in *Paediatric Short Cases for Postgraduate Examinations* by A Thomson, H Wallace and T Stephenson (Churchill Livingstone, Edinburgh, 2003).

COMMON SYNDROMES

● Neurocutaneous
● Syndromes associated with short stature
● Syndromes associated with cardiovascular disorders
● Chromosomal synrdomes
● Storage disorders

NEUROCUTANEOUS SYNDROMES

These are a group of commonly occurring exam syndromes with classical cutaneous physical signs, which should suggest the diagnosis and prompt a clinical search for associated features.

NEUROFIBROMATOSIS (VON RECKLINGHAUSEN'S DISEASE)

There are eight types described but types I and II are the most common.

Type I
● Incidence of 1 in 4000
● 90% of all neurofibromatosis cases
● Autosomal dominant, with about 50% of cases representing new mutations
● Gene locus on chromosome 17.

Clinical features   Two or more of the following are diagnostic of neurofibromatosis type I:

● six or more café-au-lait macules >5 mm in greatest diameter in prepubertal individuals and >15 mm in postpubertal individuals. Café-au-lait spots are usually present at birth
● two or more neurofibromas

- freckling in the axillary or inguinal region
- optic glioma (15%)
- two or more Lisch nodules (iris hamartomas) (found in 90% and do not occur in type II)
- distinctive osseous lesions, e.g. tibial bowing, kyphoscoliosis
- a first-degree relative with type I by the above criteria.

Associated features and complications
- Macrocephaly (46% >97th centile)
- Short stature (34% < third centile)
- Minimal learning difficulties (30%)
- Scoliosis (11.5%)
- Raised blood pressure – renal artery stenosis (2%) or phaeochromocytomas (3%)
- Malignancy (CNS, optic gliomas; schwannoma; astrocytomas [2%]; other, rhabdomyosarcoma; peripheral nerve malignancy [3%]; leukaemia)
- Seizures.

Type II
- 10% of all cases
- Autosomal dominant inheritance
- Mostly new mutations
- Gene locus on chromosome 22.

Clinical features   The diagnosis is made if the child has the following:

- bilateral acoustic neuromas
- unilateral acoustic neuroma and first-degree relative with neurofibromatosis type II
- two of the following:
  — neurofibroma
  — meningioma
  — glioma
  — schwannoma
  — juvenile posterior subscapular lenticular opacities.

Neurofibromatosis type II is also associated with café-au-lait spots but never more than six.

Conditions associated with café-au-lait spots
- Neurofibromatosis
- Tuberous sclerosis
- Fanconi's anaemia
- Ataxic telangiectasia
- Russell–Silver dwarfism
- McCune–Albright syndrome
- Bloom's syndrome
- Gaucher's disease
- Chediak–Higashi syndrome
- Normal variant.

TUBEROUS SCLEROSIS

This is a syndrome of epilepsy, mental retardation and characteristic hamartomatous lesions which develop in the skin and many other tissues.

General
- Autosomal dominant inheritance with incomplete penetrance (with a 50% recurrence risk in offspring)
- 80% are new mutations
- Prevalence of 1 in 10 000–15 000
- Gene locus on chromosomes 9 and 16.

Clinical features

Skin
- Hypopigmented macules – oval white naevi present from birth in 80% of cases
- Adenoma sebaceum – fibrous-angiomatous lesions present in 85% over the age of 5 years. Develop in the nasolabial folds and spread outwards to the cheeks in a butterfly distribution. They vary in colour from flesh to pink to yellow to brown and may coalesce to form firm plaques
- Periungual fibromata – may appear at puberty
- Shagreen patch – usually seen in the sacral region
- Café-au-lait patches – occasionally.

CNS
- Tuberous hamartomata – in the cortex and white matter in over 90%, and may calcify. A CT scan of the brain can be diagnostic
- Seizures – develop in childhood, may be myoclonic, grand mal or present as infantile spasms and are difficult to control. EEG abnormalities are common (87%) and may show a hypsarrhythmic pattern
- Mental retardation – common (40%, of whom 100% will develop seizures); of those with average intelligence about 60% will develop epilepsy
- Cerebral astrocytoma
- Malignant glioma
- Hydrocephalus.

Teeth
- Enamel hypoplasia.

Eyes
- Retinal phakomata – 40%, a yellowish multinodular cystic lesion arising from the disc or retina
- Choroidal hamartomas.

Kidney
- Renal angiomyolipomata – in 45–81%, usually multiple, benign and commonly bilateral, not palpable
- Polycystic kidneys.

Cardiac
- Rhabdomyomas – single or multiple.

Lungs
- Cystic hamartomatous nodules.

Gastrointestinal system
- Rectal polyp.

STURGE–WEBER SYNDROME

Clinical features

- Sporadic disorder of unknown aetiology present from birth.
- Haemangiomatous facial lesion in the distribution of the trigeminal nerve associated with haemangiomata of the meninges.
- The ophthalmic division of the trigeminal nerve is always involved.
- There may be involvement of the choroid of the eye with glaucoma and buphthalmos.
- Cerebral calcification may develop and has a classical appearance (double contour).
- In its most severe form it may present with:
  — epilepsy which begins in the first few months and is difficult to control
  — learning difficulties
  — hemiplegia.
- Intractable epilepsy in early infancy may benefit from hemispherectomy.
- For less severely affected children, deterioration after 5 years of age is unlikely, although seizures and learning difficulties still persist.

CAUSES OF CALCIFICATION ON SKULL X-RAY

- Tuberous sclerosis
- Arteriovenous malformation
- Sturge–Weber syndrome
- Toxoplasmosis
- Cytomegalovirus infection
- Glioma
- Astrocytoma
- Craniopharyngioma.

SHORT STATURE

The clinical approach to the child with short stature has been fully discussed in Chapter 6. In this chapter we will discuss some of the more common clinical syndromes which are associated with short stature.

PRADER–WILLI SYNDROME

- Incidence of 1 in 10 000.
- Sporadic occurrence associated with a deletion on the long arm of the paternally inherited chromosome 15 (15q11-13) or an unusual pattern of genetic inheritance known as 'imprinting'.
- Imprinting refers to gene activity that is only expressed in the copy derived from a parent of given sex. Prader–Willi and Angelman syndrome genes are separate but are both found on chromosome 15 in the 15q11–13 region. The *paternal copy* of the Prader–Willi gene and the *maternal copy* of the Angelman gene are normally active. Failure to inherit the active gene will give rise to the relevant syndrome. This can happen by two methods, either de novo deletion giving rise to a new mutation, or uniparental disomy, whereby a child inherits two copies of a region on a chromosome from one parent and none from the other. Thus, in Prader–Willi syndrome, the child will have two copies of the maternal chromosome 15q11–13, but none from the father. This can be confirmed by molecular genetic testing.

Clinical features

In infancy
- History of poor feeding
- Hypotonia in infancy.

In the older child
Face
- Narrow forehead
- Myopathic face
- Upward sloping palpebral fissures with almond-shaped eyes
- 'Carp-shaped' mouth
- Micrognathia
- Strabismus.
Skeletal
- Small hands and feet
- Clinodactyly and syndactyly (not polydactyly which is associated with Laurence–Moon–Biedl syndrome)
- Scoliosis
- Short stature.
Neurological
- Mental retardation (IQ 40–70)
- Hypotonia in infancy
- Hyperphagia with insatiable appetite after infancy which can cause severe behavioural disturbance in the quest for food.
Endocrine
- Gross obesity
- Hypogonadism – micropenis, hypoplastic scrotum, bilateral cryptorchidism
- Delayed menarche in girls
- Gonadotrophin secretion may be normal or increased
- Diabetes mellitus.

Prognosis
Life expectancy is reduced as a consequence of the obesity and associated cardiac and respiratory complications.

TURNER'S SYNDROME

- Incidence of 1 in 1500–2500 live born females (most, >95%, result in spontaneous miscarriage).
- Chromosome defect – complete or partial loss of the paternal X chromosome. Loss of the maternal X chromosome is a lethal deletion. 50% have complete loss of the X chromosome, while the remainder include mosaics involving a deletion of the short arm of the X chromosome or an isochromosome, which has two long arms and no short arms.
- The incidence does not increase with increasing maternal age.

Clinical features
The presence of ovarian dysgenesis, short stature and other dysmorphic features associated with a 45X (or XO) karyotype constitutes Turner's syndrome. It should be excluded by karyotype analysis in all girls who are short, particularly if they exhibit any of the clinical features mentioned below.

Neonatal
- Transient congenital lymphoedema present over the dorsum of the feet
- Usually small for dates.

Facial and skeletal
- Broad thorax with widely spaced nipples – 'shield chest'
- Wide carrying angle (cubitus valgus)
- Prominent ears
- Webbed neck
- Low posterior hairline
- High-arched palate
- Short fourth metacarpal and hyperconvex nails.

Neurological   Mental retardation is uncommon but a specific defect in space–form perception is often present.

Endocrine
- Increased incidence of autoimmune diseases (particularly hypothyroidism)
- Infertility and pubertal failure are the rule due to the presence of streak ovaries
- Short stature is a common problem, the mean final height being 142–147 cm +/– 12 cm.

Associated abnormalities
- A high incidence of renal abnormalities, particularly horseshoe kidneys
- Cardiac defects of which coarctation of the aorta is the commonest
- Excessive pigmented naevi.

Treatment

Growth failure
- *Growth hormone replacement therapy* – recombinant growth hormone injections increase final height by 6–8 cm. Higher doses are required than in growth hormone deficiency
- *Steroid replacement* – oxandrolone is an anabolic steroid with minimal androgenic side-effects which will increase final height when administered in low doses.

Pubertal failure
Oestrogen replacement   20% have some ovarian function and develop some signs of puberty. Most girls require oestrogen therapy at 12–13 years for the development of secondary sexual characteristics. Once puberty is initiated, cyclical therapy with oestrogen and progesterone leads to menstrual cycles. Successful pregnancies have resulted from ovum induction and in vitro fertilization.

ACHONDROPLASIA

This is the most common of the skeletal dysplasias of which there are hundreds. If bone disease is suspected as a cause of short stature (usually disproportionate), then a radiological survey of the skull, spine, pelvis and limbs is indicated.

General
- Autosomal dominant inheritance
- 50% are new mutations
- Incidence increases with increasing paternal age.

Clinical features
- Megalocephaly
- Prominent forehead
- Midfacial hypoplasia
- Short stature (mean adult height in males is 131 cm and in females 124 cm)
- Short limbs
- Thoracolumbar kyphosis.

Complications
- Hydrocephalus secondary to a narrow foramen magnum
- Spinal cord and/or root compression.

RUSSELL–SILVER SYNDROME

- Sporadic occurrence of unknown aetiology
- Prenatal onset with intrauterine growth retardation.

Clinical features
- Short stature of prenatal onset
- Limb hemihypertrophy
- Short incurved fifth finger (clinodactyly)
- Small triangular face with frontal bossing
- Café-au-lait spots
- Normal intelligence
- Bluish sclerae in early infancy.

FETAL ALCOHOL SYNDROME

Excessive alcohol intake during pregnancy is sometimes associated with the fetal alcohol syndrome.

Clinical features
- Growth retardation
- Small nose
- Maxillary hypoplasia
- Smooth philtrum
- Short, thin upper lip
- Cardiac defects in up to 70%
- Developmental delay.

SYNDROMES ASSOCIATED WITH CARDIOVASCULAR DISEASE
(see also Ch. 3)

Down's syndrome
- Atrioventricular canal defects
- Patent ductus arteriosus
- Ventricular septal defect.

Turner's syndrome
- Coarctation of the aorta
- Aortic valvular stenosis.

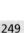
Noonan's syndrome
- Pulmonary valvular stenosis
- Peripheral pulmonary stenosis
- Atrial septal defect
- Patent ductus arteriosus
- Cardiomyopathy.

Marfan's syndrome
- Prolapsed mitral valve
- Aortic valve incompetence
- Dissecting aortic aneurysm.

Williams syndrome
- Supravalvular aortic stenosis
- Peripheral pulmonary artery stenosis
- Pulmonary valve stenosis.

Congenital rubella
- Patent ductus arteriosus
- Ventricular septal defect
- Peripheral pulmonary artery stenosis.

Ellis–van Creveld syndrome
- Atrial septal defect.

Holt–Oram syndrome
- Atrial septal defect
- Ventricular septal defect.

Maternal collagen disease
- Congenital heart block.

Pompé's disease
- Hypertrophic obstructive cardiomyopathy.

Friedreich's ataxia
- Cardiomyopathy.

Ehlers–Danlos syndrome
- Mitral valve prolapse
- Tricuspid valve prolapse.

The above list of associations either provides a clue to cardiac conditions to be excluded if you recognize the syndrome, or alternatively suggests a syndrome diagnosis if, for example, you suspect peripheral pulmonary artery stenosis.

NOONAN'S SYNDROME (BONNEVIE–ULLRICH SYNDROME)

- Previously termed male Turner's, although it occurs in both sexes, and there is a number of striking clinical differences
- Incidence of 1 in 1000–2500 live births

- Usually sporadic but occasionally familial
- Autosomal dominant inheritance with variable expressivity
- Gene locus on chromosome 12
- Normal at birth but often have feeding difficulties.

Clinical features
Facial
- Hypertelorism (75%) (see p. 238)
- Downward sloping palpebral fissures
- Epicanthic folds
- Micrognathia
- High-arched palate
- Bilateral ptosis
- Low posterior hairline
- Webbing of the neck.
Skeletal
- Short stature
- Cubitus valgus
- Shield chest
- Pectus excavatum or carinatum
- Kyphosis/scoliosis.
Endocrine
- Males – small penis, cryptorchidism
- Females – delayed menarche.
Other
- Cardiovascular – see above
- Renal abnormalities are common
- Bleeding problems occur in 20%
- Mild to moderate mental retardation in 30%
- The most striking clinical difference between Noonan's syndrome and Turner's syndrome is the presence of mental retardation and right-sided congenital heart disease in Noonan's syndrome.

WILLIAMS SYNDROME

- Occurrence is sporadic
- Aetiology is a microdeletion on chromosome 7 (elastin gene) – FISH studies.

Clinical features
Facial
- Prominent lips (and open mouth) with small teeth and snub nose
- Medial eyebrow flare
- Short palpebral fissures
- Blue eyes with stellate pattern in the iris.
Neurological
- Mild microcephaly
- Mild mental retardation (average IQ 56).
Skeletal
- Mild prenatal growth deficiency
- Hypoplastic nails.
Other
- Outgoing and loquacious with a 'cocktail party' personality
- Transient neonatal hypercalcaemia occasionally

- Cardiovascular (see above)
- Renal artery stenosis
- Bladder diverticula
- Partial anodontia or microdontia.

ELLIS–VAN CREVELD SYNDROME

- Autosomal dominant inheritance.

Clinical features
- Postaxial polydactyly
- Micromelic dwarfism (shortening is most marked in the distal half of each limb)
- Congenital heart disease (see above)
- Ectodermal dysplasia.

HOLT–ORAM SYNDROME

- Autosomal dominant inheritance.

Clinical features
- Congenital anomalies of the thumb and radius
- Atrial or ventricular septal defects.

CHROMOSOMAL SYNDROMES

DOWN'S SYNDROME (TRISOMY 21)

- Incidence of 1 in 650 live births
- Incidence increases with increasing maternal age
- Commonest autosomal trisomy. Extra chromosome 21 may result from non-disjunction (94%), translocation (5%) or mosaicism (1%)
- Commonest cause of severe mental retardation.

Clinical features
A child with Down's syndrome is common in exams and therefore you will be expected to know a lot about it. The children are usually very cooperative and enjoy the extra attention lavished upon them. A whole short case may focus, for example, just on the hand in Down's syndrome, so that to score well you need to be well prepared. Many of the clinical features of Down's syndrome are well known and in this chapter we have focused on a few areas which tend to be commonly explored by examiners.

Common features in the newborn 89% of a series of 48 newborns with Down's syndrome had six or more of the following:

- hypotonia – 80%
- poor Moro reflex – 85%
- hyperflexibility of joints – 80%
- excess skin on back of neck – 80%
- flat facial profile – 90%
- slanted palpebral fissures – 80%

Clinical paediatrics for postgraduate exams

- anomalous auricles – 60%
- dysplasia of pelvis – 70%
- dysplasia of midphalanx of fifth finger – 60%
- single palmar crease – 45%.

The head and neck

- Flat occiput and third fontanelle
- Round face
- Epicanthic folds
- Brushfield spots in the iris
- Cataracts
- Refractive errors
- Strabismus
- Protruding tongue (due to relatively small mouth, not macroglossia)
- Small ears.

The hand

- Short metacarpals and phalanges (small and broad hands)
- Transverse palmar crease (45%)
- Fifth finger
  — hypoplasia or absence of the middle phalanx (60%)
  — clinodactyly (50%)
  — a single crease (40%)
- Hyperextensibility
- Dermatoglyphics (for an excellent introduction to this important area, see Appendix 1 of *Developmental Defects and Syndromes* by M A Salmon (H M + M Publishers, Aylesbury, 1978).
  — Palms
    — distal position of palmar axial triradius
    — a loop in the hypothenar region (Fig. 11.6)
    — a loop in the third interdigital area
  — Fingers
    — ulnar loops are common
    — radial loops may be found on digits IV and V.

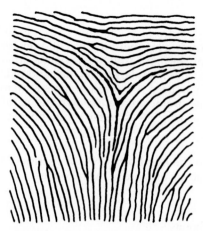

Fig. 11.6 Triradius – the meeting of three dermal ridge patterns. (Reproduced with permission from Forfar J O, Arneil G C (eds) 1984 Textbook of Paediatrics, 3rd edn. Churchill Livingstone, Edinburgh.)

Common associations
- Duodenal stenosis or atresia
- Pyloric stenosis
- Small bowel atresias
- Hirschsprung's disease
- Anal atresia
- Biliary atresia
- Recurrent respiratory infections
- Hearing impairment from recurrent secretory otitis media
- Visual impairment from squints or cataracts
- Severe learning difficulties
- Short stature
- Increased risk of leukaemia
- Risk of atlantoaxial instability (rare)
- Thyroid disorders (more commonly hypothyroidism)
- Alzheimer's disease
- Males – hypogonadism and infertility is universal
- Females – delayed menarche, secondary amenorrhoea and premature menopause are common.

STORAGE DISORDERS

MUCOPOLYSACCHARIDOSES

These are a group of inherited progressive, multisystem disorders of glycosaminoglycan metabolism which are not uncommonly seen in paediatric examinations.

Hurler's syndrome (MPS1)
- Inheritance is autosomal recessive
- Diagnosis is by finding excess secretion of dermatan and heparan sulphates in the urine
- Normal appearance at birth; usually present with developmental delay at 6–12 months
- Poor prognosis with death from cardiorespiratory complications by the end of the first decade.

Clinical features
Eyes
- Corneal clouding
- Retinal pigmentation
- Glaucoma.

Skin
- Coarse facies with increasing age
- Large tongue and thick lips
- Hypertrichosis.

Skeletal
- Thickened skull
- Limitation of joint movement with the development of claw hand
- Broad ribs
- Thoracolumbar kyphosis
- Bone changes known as dysostosis multiplex
- Normal linear growth for the first year followed by the development of short stature.

Heart
- Valvular lesions
- Cardiac failure.

Neurological
- Developmental regression.

Other
- Hepatosplenomegaly
- Umbilical and inguinal herniae
- Carpel tunnel syndrome
- Conductive deafness.

Hunter's syndrome

Similar features to Hurler's syndrome, but the course is more benign and inheritance is X-linked recessive. There is no corneal clouding. Diagnosis is confirmed by the presence of excess dermatan and heparan sulphates in the urine.

SUMMARY OF EXAMINATION OF CHILD WITH DYSMORPHIC FEATURES

INSPECTION

Head

Does the *size* look normal and in proportion to the body? Micro/macrocephaly (plot OFC, largest of three measurements, on centile chart)

Is the *shape* normal?

Are the *sutures* normal?

Eyes

Is the face symmetrical? Do the eyes look abnormally close together or far apart, e.g. Apert's, Crouzon's, Carpenter's?

Know how to test for hypo/hypertelorism (see p. 240)

Microphthalmus or buphthalmos?

Epicanthic folds

Palpebral fissures

Synophrys, coloboma, ptosis

Orbital ridges, shallow or prominent

Corneal clouding

Blue sclera

Heterochromia iridae

Ears

Low-set? Know how to test for low-set ears (see text)

Shape, size, auricular tags, accessory auricles

Look with auriscope if necessary

Face

Shape, symmetry

Maxillary/mandibular hypoplasia?

Gums hypertrophied or ulcerated?

Cleft lip or palate? High-arched palate?

Prominent lips

Pallor, cyanosis

Macroglossia, mouth ulcers, oral thrush

Teeth, numbers, caries, pigmented

Tonsils

Hands

Simian creases

Brachydactyly, clinodactyly, poldactyly, syndactyly, arachnodactyly

Broad thumbs, absent thumbs/radii

Skin

Alopecia, hirsutism

Hyper/hypopigmentation

Genitalia

Cryptorchidism, hypospadias, micropenis

Once you have pieced together the dysmorphic features, ask the examiner if you can now go on and examine the relevant system, e.g. cardiovascular system in Down's syndrome.

The neonate

12

Neonatal examination is important for several reasons.

- To identify any consequences of the birth itself, e.g. cephalhaematoma
- To assess adaptation to extrauterine life
- To assess gestational age and confirm the maturity of the baby
- To detect any congenital anomalies identifiable at this early stage and discuss their appropriate management with the parents
- To recognize if the baby is ill and requires transfer to the neonatal unit for further management.

In the exam situation the most likely reason to be asked to examine a neonate is in the context of ex-prematurity or if the baby has a congenital abnormality.

EXAMINATION

GENERAL OBSERVATIONS

Growth and nutritional status
- Is the baby thriving?
- Plot the weight, length and head circumference on a growth chart appropriate for the baby's age, sex and ethnic group.

Was this infant born prematurely?

Is he/she dysmorphic?
- Dysmorphology is much more difficult in the neonate than in the older child and only definite abnormalities should be noted (see Ch. 11). 'Soft signs' are usually because he/she looks like his/her parents!

Skin

Colour
- Pallor
- Plethora – think of small for gestational age and infant of diabetic mother
- Jaundice is very common in >60% of term babies
  — clinical jaundice is when bilirubin reaches 80–100 mmol/L
  — need to know management
- Cyanosis – peripheral cyanosis of the hands and feet is common on the first day. For central/persistent cyanosis see Chapter 4
  — traumatic cyanosis from a cord around the baby's neck or from a face presentation associated with petechiae over the head and neck but the tongue is pink
- Chronic meconium staining of the nails and the umbilical stump.

Rashes

Urticaria neonatorum (Erythema toxicum)
● Very common benign, self-resolving rash appearing at 2–3 days of age usually on the trunk
● White/yellow pinpoint papules at the centre of an erythematous base. The papules are sterile and contain eosinophils.

Birth marks

Mongolian blue spot
● Blue/black macule, sometimes multiple
● Lumbosacral region or buttocks
● Majority of Oriental, Asian, African and Carribbean infants
● Most fade spontaneously.

Stork bites
● Red macules – superficial capillary haemangioma
● Often on the nape of the neck or the forehead
● Those on the forehead fade spontaneously, those on the neck fade a little and become covered with hair.

Naevi

Strawberry naevus (cavernous haemangioma)
● Not present at birth but usually appears within the first month
● More common in preterm infants
● Increases in size until 3–9 months of age, then gradually regresses
● No treatment required unless it interferes with vision or the airway
● Ulceration or haemorrhage may occur
● Thrombocytopenia may occur with large lesions and may be treated with systemic steroids or alpha-interferon.

Port-wine stain (naevus flamus)
● Red to purple flat lesion
● Vascular malformation of the capillaries in the dermis
● Can occur anywhere
● May be unilateral and, rarely, occurs along the distribution of the trigeminal nerve. May be associated with intracranial vascular anomalies (Sturge–Weber syndrome)
● Does not resolve
● Disfiguring lesions can be improved with laser therapy.

Maturity You must be familiar with the general principles of the Dubowitz examination, although you would not be expected to have memorized every detail. You are unlikely to see the thin gelatinous skin of a newly born premature infant. Postmature infants often have wrinkled or desquamating skin, particularly over the creases of the hands; desquamation may also occur with staphylococcal infections.

Having taken a look at the infant overall, the easiest way of examining the newborn is from head to toe, rather than by system. Particular points to note in the neonate will be emphasized, and material included in the chapters on individual systems will not be duplicated.

FACE

● Flaring of the alar nasi is a sign of respiratory distress
● Look for bruising and forceps marks

- Marked facial asymmetry suggests facial nerve palsy
- Look at ears for maturity, bruising, pre-auricular tags and position (see Ch. 11 for definition of low-set ears).

EYES

- Look for hypertelorism and the angle of the palpebral fissures (see Ch. 11). Do not comment unless definitely abnormal.
- Subconjunctival haemorrhages frequently occur following completely normal birth.
- Faintly blue sclera are normal in the newborn so do not assume osteogenesis imperfecta without supporting evidence.
- A newborn term infant should fix, follow and turn to light but may also have a non-paralytic strabismus. This is unusual after 3 months and definitely abnormal after 6 months.
- Congenital ptosis may be unilateral or bilateral and may be associated with an inability to look up. Ptosis is not often a sign of myasthenia in the newborn (unlike the older child).
- The pupils are reactive from 29–32 weeks' gestation. Different-sized pupils are a normal variant (physiological anisocoria) provided both pupils respond normally to light. A blind eye will show a consensual light reflex but no direct light reflex.
- Each eye may have a different coloured iris (heterochromiairidia) and this may be a normal variant or a feature of Waardenburg's syndrome.
- Red reflex – if the infant's eyes are open, shine an ophthalmoscope on each eye from about 15 cm away. Trying to force the eyes open will make the baby cry and will not impress the examiners. Two tricks to persuade a baby to open his/her eyes are to give him/her something to suck or to ask the mother to hold her baby facing over her shoulder. If the red reflex is absent, or partly obscured, there may be a cataract, and formal ophthalmoscopy is indicated at the end of the examination. This involves:

Inspection of the cornea   Do this still from 15 cm away with the ophthalmoscope lens set to 'red 10'.

White pupil and absent red reflex of cataract
- Majority are inherited (usually autosomal dominant)
- Intrauterine rubella
- Galactosaemia (not present at birth but may appear by second week)
- Lowe's syndrome.

Hazy broad cornea   (>1 cm diameter) of congenital glaucoma. Buphthalmos is tremendous enlargement of the eyeball as an end-stage of the disease.
- Majority inherited (autosomal recessive)
- Intrauterine rubella.

Coloboma
- CHARGE association
  — Coloboma
  — Heart disease
  — Atresia choanae
  — Retarded growth
  — Genital abnormality or hypogonadism
  — Ear anomalies and/or deafness
- Associated with deformities of the ears and vertebrae (Goldenhar's syndrome).

Conjunctivitis
- Viral, bacterial or chlamydial.

Dermoid   The eye is a favourite site, usually where the cornea joins the sclera.

Fundoscopy   Offer to attempt this, although it is unlikely to be taken up unless the infant's pupils have already been dilated with mydriatics. In this case, there is probably one of the following:

- retinopathy of prematurity (retrolental fibroplasia) – this causes proliferation of new vessels and eventually cicatricial fibrosis and retinal detachment
- chorioretinitis (posterior uveitis) – this occurs as a result of intrauterine infection
- retinal haemorrhages – these occur in 20% of all newborns following a normal delivery.

Skull (See Ch. 8)

Remember that sutures may be wider or overriding in the first few days after birth and the anterior fontanelle may be 1–5 cm in diameter. Parietal foramina may occur and are bilateral and familial.

- Fetal scalp electrodes may cause a bruise or small laceration.
- Caput is pitting oedema and may extend across suture lines.
- Cephalhaematoma is a tense collection of blood and is bounded by suture lines. Cephalhaematoma should not be confused with cranial meningocoele or encephalo-meningocoele. These are usually midline, occipital, soft to palpation, and the bony defect of a cranium bifidum should be apparent.
- Feel for a reservoir or the catheter of a ventriculoperitoneal shunt, especially if hydrocephalus is obvious, but leave measurement of the occipito-frontal circumference (OFC) to the end of the examination.
- Scaphocephaly (literally 'boat shaped', i.e. long and narrow) is common in 'ex-prems' (up to school age) and plagiocephaly is common and usually benign in term infants.

Mouth

Normal variants.

- Incisor teeth
- Epithelial 'pearls' along the midline of the palate
- Short lingual frenum (not frenulum which is between upper gum and lip). Only very rarely requires surgery for interference with tongue growth or speech.

Check the hard palate   Feel along the hard palate with the pulp of your little finger. A cleft palate may be submucous and not visible. Offer to look in the mouth with a bright torch (not an ophthalmoscope which is too dim) and wooden spatula. If the examiners agree to this, there is likely to be one of the following:

- cleft of soft palate – look for micrognathia suggesting Pierre–Robin sequence. A slanting lower jaw may also reflect intrauterine posture or oligohydramnios (fetal inertia syndrome, in which there may also be talipes equinovarus, camptodactyly and even arthrogryposis)
- ranula – a cyst in the floor of the mouth arising from the salivary ducts

- haemangioma of the tongue
- bifid tongue
- tongue fasciculation in spinal muscular atrophy (see Ch. 8).

If there is a white covering of the tongue or buccal mucosa, it may be candida but ask if the infant has just been fed.

NECK

Swellings occurring in the newborn are:

Midline
- goitre
- thymic cyst
- thyroglossal duct cyst (moves with tongue movement)
- epidermoid cyst.

Lateral
- sternomastoid 'tumour' – fibrous nodule midway along the muscle which causes torticollis. Usually does not appear until 2 weeks of age and most resolve by 8–10 weeks with physiotherapy. Associated with breech delivery and congenital dislocation of the hips and talipes equinovarus
- cystic hygroma – benign lymphangioma
- branchial cyst – vestigial remnant of branchial arch during ontogeny
- ectopic thyroid.

Tumours and abscesses in the neck are extremely rare in the newborn period.

Now undress the baby except for the nappy, always remembering to observe the breathing rate and pattern before disturbing him/her (see Ch. 5).

CHEST AND HEART

Inspection
Observation is much more important in assessing the respiratory system than palpation, percussion or auscultation. Watching and listening to the baby's breathing will reveal most things.

- Respiratory distress
  — tachypnoea, grunting, flaring of the alar nasi and intercostal or subcostal recession may suggest respiratory, cardiac or neurological problems
  — remember, abnormalities of the airway, the cardiovascular system, the chest wall, the muscles, nerves, spinal cord or brain may all create respiratory distress as well as lung pathology
- Stridor
  — most commonly due to laryngomalacia
  — subglottic stenosis should be considered in an 'ex-prem'
- Chronic lung disease
  — hyperinflation
  — may have chronic oxygen requirement.

Palpation
- Pulses – feel for both brachial pulses but leave femoral pulses to the end of the examination.

Auscultation

- This gives little information about the respiratory system in the newborn but is usually performed front and back bilaterally while listening to the cardiac sounds.
- Normal newborn respiration is quiet, effortless and predominantly diaphragmatic. There is more abdominal than chest movement.
- Innocent murmurs are much commoner in young babies than older children and the second heart sound is much more difficult to assess.

HANDS

Look for:

- palmar creases
- number of digits
- syndactyly
- clinodactyly
- paronychia if present.

ABDOMEN

Inspection

The abdomen is usually protruberant (especially after a feed!). Examine the umbilical stump (if present) for:

- infection
- two umbilical arteries
- exomphalos
- granuloma
- look for hernia – an umbilical hernia is particularly common in African infants.

Palpation

Regurgitation frequently occurs and is not abnormal. It is normal to be able to palpate in the newborn:

- tip of the spleen
- 1 cm soft liver edge
- lower poles of both kidneys
- bladder – a bladder to the umbilicus should suggest spina bifida or damage to the central nervous system.

Leave inspection of the groins, genitalia and hips until the end of the examination.

NERVOUS SYSTEM

The commonest pitfall in the neonatal neurological examination is that the responses vary with wakefulness, gestation and if the head is not in the midline. A brief description is given below but more detail can be found in the neurology chapter.

Cranial nerves

Examination of the face, eyes and tongue has already been described. Most babies will have cried at some point during the above sequence and a feeble cry or persistent irritability and a high-pitched cry may be obvious.

- Glabella tap – a persistent blink response is normal and present from 32–34 weeks' gestation.
- Rooting reflex – stroke the cheek and the infant turns his/her head to that side.
- Sucking reflex – elicited by pressure on the hard palate with a finger while examining for a cleft.

Assessment of hearing and vision are discussed in Chapter 9.

Posture
- Normal – flexed 'fetal' or frog-like when supine.
- Hypotonia – fully abducted hips in a term infant. Premature infants are normally 'floppy' by comparison. Other features of hypotonia are:
  — abnormal head lag during 'pull to sit'
  — a tendency to slip through the examiner's grasp in vertical suspension, the candidate grasping the infant under each axilla
  — a 'rag doll' flexion of the spine in ventral suspension.
- Head lag – most term infants have no head lag by 3 months and head lag is definitely abnormal by 5 months.
- Ventral suspension – most infants have a straight back by 6 weeks.
- Prone – most term infants cannot maintain 'head up' at 90° until 8–10 weeks. If present at birth, this implies hypertonicity, as does opisthotonus and an extensor posture rather than the flexed 'fetal' posture.

These developmental attainments do not obey postconceptional age, insofar as neurodevelopment is accelerated in the premature infant compared to in utero, but they are still likely to occur at a somewhat later postnatal age than in the term infant.

Tone and power
These are assessed from resistance to undressing and during assessment of posture. Assess flexor recoil and compare sides.

Reflexes
Deep tendon reflexes are extremely difficult to elicit in the newborn, except perhaps the knee jerks. A few beats of ankle clonus may be present in the normal infant. Primitive cranial nerve reflexes have been mentioned above. Other primitive reflexes are:

- grasp reflex – hands and feet grasp in response to pressure. Normally lost by 2 months.
- stepping reflex – child steps if lowered onto a hard surface. Normally lost by 2 months.
- asymmetrical tonic neck reflex – in response to rotation of the head to one side, the arm on that side extends and the other flexes. Difficult to perform properly as the infant must start in a position with his/her head in the midline and the limbs held symmetrically. Normally lost by 6 months. An abnormal tonic neck reflex, say the right arm extends less on rotation of the head to the right than the left arm does on extension of the head to the left, implies an abnormality of the right side in this example.
- Moro reflex – must start from a symmetrical position. On dropping the head 2–3 cm, the upper limbs should abduct and extend symmetrically. An asymmetric response again implies a hemiparesis which may be central (e.g. cerebral palsy) or peripheral (e.g. brachial plexus birth injury). Normally lost by 6 months.

- plantar reflex – bilaterally upgoing until about 12 months.
- Galant reflex – in ventral suspension, stroking one side of the spine causes flexion of the spine on that side. May not disappear until 5 years old.

These reflexes may persist until a slightly later postnatal age in the premature infant but again development is accelerated ahead of the postconceptual age.

COMPLETING THE EXAMINATION

We have suggested that a number of tasks be left until the end of the examination as the child may find them unpleasant. Do not forget to examine, or offer to examine, the following:

Femoral pulses   In a baby, it is often easier to feel the femoral pulses with your thumbs and this is permissible.

Groins   Check for herniae in either sex. Inguinal hernia is more common in preterms, boys and on the right side.

Genitalia
- Increased pigmentation – abnormal in both sexes unless Asian or Afro-Caribbean baby
- Boys
  — epispadias – very rare
  — hypospadias – glandular is relatively common; penile or perineal is exceedingly rare
  — small penis of hypopituitarism
  — scrotum for descent of testes and hydrocoeles
- Girls
  — size of clitoris
  — labial fusion
  — a clear vaginal discharge and blood are both normal in the immediate newborn period.

Hips (see Ch. 10)

Turn the infant over.

Anus, sacrum and spine   Run a finger along the spine, coccyx to occiput. A lumbo-sacral dimple is less likely to be benign if:

- it is high
- it is away from the midline
- the base is not visible
- it is associated with hairy naevus or a palpable defect in the spine
- there is weakness of the legs or a patulous anus.

Occipito-frontal circumference
Fundoscopy
Blood pressure

COMMON LONG CASE

THE 'EX-PREM'

Graduates of the neonatal unit are common and many exhibit persistent stigmata from their admission and some have chronic diseases or handicaps. They therefore make ideal cases for the membership or DCH exams.

HISTORY

Great attention must obviously be paid to the history of pregnancy and the perinatal period, and most of the pertinent questions have been referred to in earlier chapters (see Ch. 2 'The long case', and Ch. 8 'The developmental examination').

Pre-natal
● What was the mother's health like during pregnancy?
● Did she have any infections/hypertension/gestational diabetes?
● What was her antibody status (rubella)?
● How many previous pregnancies and what was the outcome?

Perinatal
● Was the onset of labour spontaneous?
● When did her membranes rupture in relation to the birth?
● How premature was the baby?
● Was the mother transferred in utero or was the baby collected by a 'flying squad'? In either case, the mother may have had to spend long periods away from her kin
● Was immediate resuscitation required in the delivery room?
● Did the baby receive oxygen or ventilation and, if so, for how long?
● Did the baby require a chest drain?
● How long did the baby spend in NICU?
● Did the baby receive nasogastric (expressed breast milk or a premature formula) or parenteral nutrition?
● Did the baby have one or more lumbar punctures? Why?
● Was there phototherapy or an exchange transfusion?

Postnatal
● What support did the family have when the infant was finally allowed home?
● Did the baby require to go home on home oxygen?
● Has the baby been fully immunised?

Impact on the family
● Try to define the impact of a premature birth on the parents and the family.
● Was there a delay before the parents could hold their new baby?
● Did they 'live in' for a long period and how did they organize transport, work and care of the other children?
● Did they have fears about death and handicap and do these persist or have they been allayed?

EXAMINATION

A detailed examination following the guidelines given above must be carried out. Developmental assessment, including vision and hearing, is crucial. The following features are particularly common in infants who have been born prematurely:

● proportionate small stature
● scaphocephaly
● skin stigmata
  — pneumothorax scars
  — scars at sites of venous and arterial cannulation

— scars on the heels from repeated 'autolet' stabs
   — burns from extravasation of hypertonic fluids (e.g. parenteral nutrition fluids or sodium bicarbonate)
   — thoracic or abdominal surgical scars
   — bronzing from recent phototherapy

- stridor or tracheostomy following subglottic stenosis
- hyperinflation, recession and tachypnoea of BPD. The infant may still be receiving oxygen by mask or nasal cannulae
- patent ductus arteriosus
- hydrocephalus and/or ventriculoperitoneal (VP) or ventriculoatrial (VA) shunt following periventricular haemorrhage. VP shunts block more commonly but VA shunts require more frequent revision as the child grows. Infection rates are about the same
- retinopathy of prematurity – originally thought to have been explained by excessively high oxygen tension in arterial blood (15 kPa) but it is now clear that the aetiology is multifactorial.

DISCUSSION

You would be expected to be familiar with at least some of the many studies of long term follow-up of low birthweight infants, particularly with reference to:

- neurological development
- physical handicap, including impaired hearing and vision
- chronic lung disease
- sudden infant death.

The oral examination

13

In the oral section of the MRCPCH examination, candidates will meet a pair of examiners, each of whom will ask questions for 10 minutes. The examiners are advised to cover at least four separate subjects during the 20 minutes. There are a number of areas which examiners are discouraged from exploring, in particular factual recall and data interpretation since these have been tested in the written section of the Part II examination.

Examiners are encouraged to base their assessment of candidates on knowledge of four areas of the structured viva. The viva topics are divided into two sections. The examiners are encouraged by the RCPCH to test all candidates on the management of acute emergencies and communication skills/ethics. At least two other topics will be selected, one from Section A and one from Section B:

- *Section A*
  1. Compulsory – management of emergencies
  plus one from:
  2. Diagnostic problems
  3. Planning management of chronic disease
  4. Recent literature including new developments.
- *Section B*
  1. Compulsory – communication skills and ethics
  plus one from:
  2. Physiology and pathophysiology
  3. Psychology; social and behavioural paediatrics
  4. Clinical research or audit/resource management/statistics.

Child abuse is an example of the social side of paediatrics which is frequently asked about. Examiners are requested that one question relate to neonatology.

Within these broad headings, examiners can usually find some category into which they can slip their favourite questions. Examiners are not supposed to ask about their own specialist field but frequently do. The eight topics listed above could embrace all of the following:

- understanding of basic principles of physiology, biochemistry, applied anatomy and applied pharmacology
- simple statistics
- audit/resource management
- ability to manage acute and emergency clinical situations
- ability to plan investigations and therapeutic regimens for complex clinical problems and chronic diseases
- knowledge of the natural history of diseases
- ability to recognize, investigate and treat conditions unlikely to be seen in the clinical examination

- appreciation of social, psychological and environmental factors as they affect illness and health
- child psychiatry
- appreciation of the importance of communication with patients and their relatives
- ethics
- recent developments – including literature.

Candidates often seem bemused by the simplest questions on basic statistics. A working statistical knowledge is essential for reading the paediatric literature, keeping up to date and incorporating your reading into evidence-based practice. This is why the College emphasizes statistics in the viva. Of course, examiners are also reminded that if the candidate knows absolutely nothing about a topic, they should move on to another question, but if you do not know anything about that either, then you are in trouble. Remember that a candidate will fail if he or she records three bare fails or lower in the eight mark sheets, or if he or she records two outright fails or lower from separate examiners (see Ch. 1). Therefore, the viva is no longer a 'soft' option. If both viva examiners score you outright fails, you fail the whole exam irrespective of how well you have done in the long and short cases. Hence, a little preparation on basic statistics, even for the non-numerate doctor, may be wise.

A basic syllabus for statistics at MRCPCH level would include:

Descriptive statistics

- Mean, median and mode ('measuring the middle' – measures of central tendency)
- Standard deviation, standard error of the mean, centiles, interquartile range, minimum and maximum ('measuring the variation' – measures of dispersion)
- Normal and skewed distributions
- Qualitative data (counted or categorical) and quantitative data (measured).

Hypothesis testing (comparative testing between two groups and looking for association between two variables)

- The null hypothesis
- The concept of statistical significance
- Paired and unpaired tests (e.g. paired and unpaired *t*-tests to compare two normally distributed samples)
- Parametric and non-parametric methods (e.g. Mann–Whitney *U*-test for two unpaired non-normal samples and Wilcoxon's signed rank test for two paired non-normal samples)
- The principles of randomized controlled trials and possible sources of bias
- Chi-squared test for qualitative data; often used to see if actual counts comply with those expected on theoretical grounds but also to test the null hypothesis (here the 'theoretical' prediction is no difference between the groups)
- Some concept of correlation and regression.

Useful simple books include:

Broughton Pipkin F 1984 Medical statistics made easy. Churchill Livingstone, Edinburgh
Castle W M, North P M 1995 Statistics in small doses, 3rd edn. Churchill Livingstone, Edinburgh

Some candidates are even more ignorant of ethics and child psychiatry than they are of statistics. Some guidance on child psychiatric topics is provided in Chapter 1. You should practise, before the exam, dissecting out the ethical principles in common paediatric dilemmas.

- Conflict of parental autonomy and the doctor's role of doing most good
- Issues of informed consent and the developmental age of the patient ('Gillick competence')
- The balance of the burden to the child of intensive care versus the chances of extending life with a quality that the average person would like to live
- The five situations in which the RCPCH considers withholding or withdrawing life-prolonging treatment might be considered in the UK currently:
  — the brain dead child
  — the persistent vegetative state
  — the 'no chance' situation
  — the 'no purpose' situation
  — the 'unbearable' situation.

The examiners don't expect detailed moral philosophical jargon, nor are they testing the candidate's own religious beliefs or whether the candidate would make the moral choice prevalent in the UK (which might be affected by cultural and economic differences). However, candidates should be aware of the difficulties related to confidentiality, autonomy, avoiding harm and maximizing benefit, and fairness and justice in a health service with finite resources.

It is quite impossible and unrealistic for you to expect to know everything about anything that may be asked in the oral. On the contrary, we would advise you to select topics which you consider a reasonable examiner might *require* you to have a good working knowledge of. For example, we have listed a few subjects which we consider examiners might expect a candidate to have a comprehensive understanding of:

- the physiological basis of cyanosis
- the side-effects of long-term steroid use
- the causes of hyponatraemia and hyperkalaemia
- the management of an acute asthmatic attack or stridor
- the management of diabetic ketoacidosis
- the investigation of short stature
- the investigation of failure to thrive
- the performance of a sweat test
- the recommended immunization schedule and established contraindications.

These are examples of topics which examiners might reasonably expect a worthy candidate to be able to cope with sensibly. Most candidates do not fail on the oral alone; it is the short cases that are at the heart of the exam. However, marks can be lost in the oral by a poorly prepared candidate.

Good preparation obviously requires a sound understanding of the kind of topics mentioned above, but also includes a broad knowledge of issues in child health which are currently being debated. The annotations in *Archives of Disease in Childhood* are essential reading. This journal is distributed to all paediatricians who are members of the Royal College of Paediatrics and Child Health and is thus widely read by examiners. Other useful sources of information include *Current Paediatrics, Current Opinions in Paediatrics, British Medical Journal* and the *Lancet*.

SOME USEFUL GENERAL ADVICE

- Dress smartly – rightly or wrongly examiners expect the candidates to be well turned out.
- Treat the examiners with respect. Don't look at your feet; make eye contact and speak clearly.
- Sit up straight in the chair and do not slouch or fiddle with your hands. Sit on your hands if you are prone to fidgeting.
- Do not argue with the examiners even if you are certain you are right. Politely say: 'That was my understanding of the subject' or 'That was what I was taught at the hospital where I worked.'
- *Answer the question asked*, and if you don't understand it, ask the examiner to repeat it.
- Try to think through your answer and frame it in some system of classification before you open your mouth, rather than saying the first thing that comes into your head. Start with simple or common investigations and diagnoses. Consider the two examples below:

Example A

Examiner: 'Tell me about the causes of bruising?'

Candidate 1: 'Haemophilia, warfarin overdose, meningococcal disease, thrombocytopenia…etc.'

Candidate 2: 'Bruising can be spontaneous or traumatic. Spontaneous bruising can arise due to problems with any of the three elements of the blood coagulation system: low or abnormal platelets; low clotting factors; abnormal blood vessel endothelium. All are rare, but commoner examples of these in childhood would be idiopathic thrombocytopenic purpura or von Willebrand's disease; haemophilia or vitamin K deficiency; meningococcal septicaemia.'

If you were the examiner, who would you give the better mark to? Both candidates have given similar lists of differential diagnoses but who is the more organized in their thinking and who is less likely to miss a diagnosis by working logically in clinic or A&E rather than relying on long lists.

Example B

Examiner: 'Tell me how you would investigate jaundice in a 7-year-old?'

Candidate 1: 'Blood for bilirubin, ultrasound scan, FBC, urine…etc.'

Candidate 2: 'Jaundice can be conjugated (usually obstruction) or unconjugated (usually haemolysis) or mixed (usually hepatitis). There may be clues from history or examination, e.g. pallor, splenomegaly in haemolytic jaundice; green/brown skin rather than yellow in unconjugated jaundice. Investigation starts with examination of the stools (pale in obstruction) and urinalysis; there is no urobilinogen in the urine in obstructive jaundice but the urine is darker because of increased excretion of conjugated bilirubin. I would then undertake blood tests for conjugated and unconjugated serum bilirubin and for a full blood count and film. To avoid the child having repeat venepuncture, I would take blood at the same time, for clotting screen, blood group and Coombs' test and save a heparinized and clotted sample. However, the relevance of these further blood investigations, and whether to proceed to other tests, would depend on the results of the initial tests.'

If you were the examiner, who would you give the better mark to? Both have given similar lists of tests but who has shown that they understand the underlying principles?

These two examples may appear contrived, but real candidates do come out with long lists, usually with the rarest and most irrelevant answers first, and then omit the most usual diagnosis or test relevant to the UK. 'Common things are common.'

- Do not be afraid to say that you don't know. In a sense the examiners want to find out what you do know rather than what you don't. However, if you decline a question which is considered basic, e.g. emergency management or immunizations, you will not do well!
- Avoid mentioning topics or diseases about which you know nothing whatsoever; alternatively, you can try to lead the examiners into areas with which you are familiar.
- Be prepared for the examiner who asks you what you would like to talk about.
- Don't rely on encouraging or discouraging non-verbal clues from the examiners, as they are usually not forthcoming.
- Do not confabulate!

The oral examination

Appendix
Useful equipment for the clinical examination

The clinical centres for the MRCPCH and DCH will provide standard equipment appropriate to the examination but recommend that all candidates should bring their own stethoscope. Candidates attempting the clinical examination, and especially the short cases, are often unsure of which items of equipment to bring with them. In theory, everything which might conceivably be required should be provided by the examination centre, but this equipment will not be as familiar as your own and unnecessary delays may occur while it is located by the exam organizers. There is a need to strike a balance between adequate equipment and pockets that are bulging with everything but the kitchen sink! It is perfectly reasonable to carry a small case or bag with you into the examination, containing equipment to aid physical examination and developmental examination.

Equipment which we suggest you bring yourself
- Paediatric (not neonatal size) stethoscope with bell and diaphragm
- Watch with a second hand
- A bright pen torch with fresh batteries, which can be used for assessing corneal reflections, pupillary reactions and transillumination
- Ophthalmoscope with fresh batteries and interchangeable oroscope head. Using an unfamiliar ophthalmoscope or one with weak batteries will not be an asset when you are nervous in the short case situation
- Cotton wool
- Tape measure
- A hat pin with a red head for testing visual fields in an older child. It is stipulated that if the use of a pin is necessary for sensory examination, this will be provided by the examining centre
- 'Hundreds and thousands' and 'raisins' to test pincer grasp and visual acuity in a young child
- A small red cube for testing grasp and visual fixation in a young infant
- A small toy which has a rattle (hearing assessment), colour (visual assessment) and which can be grasped by the child. Three bricks of different colours but standard size (approx. 1.5 inches) are useful
- Picture cards (or a book from the 'Ladybird' series) which show:
  — simple pictures of animals, etc. for object recognition or hearing assessment

— situation pictures, e.g. the postman delivering parcels for a child's birthday, to test comprehension and speech
If the book contains text, make sure you know the appropriate reading age of the material
● A red woolly ball (for visual acuity in the young infant, see Table 8.2)
● Pen and paper to encourage the child to scribble, copy or draw.

Probably the strongest argument for collecting this equipment together is that this will encourage you to use it in your preparation. Strange though it may seem, we have frequently taught candidates 1 week before the clinicals who examine the chest, heart and abdomen perfectly but are completely inept with an ophthalmoscope or a cover test! This set of aids to the examination should not be assembled the night before. They must be collected and used repeatedly before the examination until you are familiar with the purpose of each item and the age range for which it is appropriate.

Index

Index

Index